RAISING GIRLS: DEVOTIONAL FOR MOM

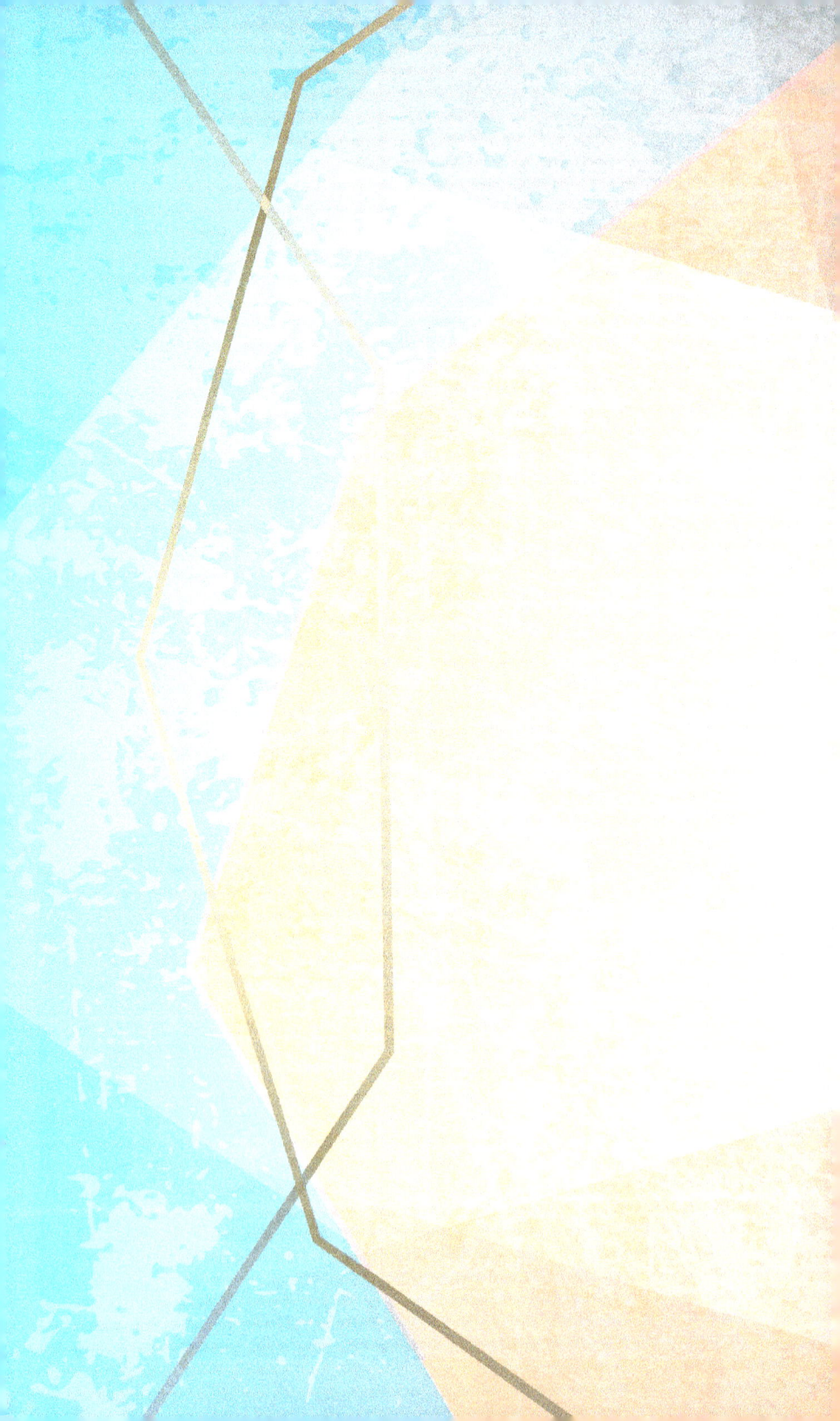

RAISING GIRLS
DEVOTIONAL FOR MOM

60 Days of Uplifting, Faith-Filled Wisdom

CECILY DICKEY

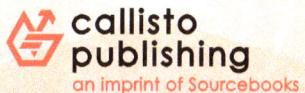

Copyright © 2022 by Callisto Publishing LLC
Cover and internal design © 2022 by Callisto Publishing LLC
All images used under license © Shutterstock.
Author photo courtesy of Jessica Dyck
Interior and Cover Designer: Alan Carr
Art Producer: Samantha Ulban
Editor: Carolyn Abate
Production Editor: Jael Fogle
Production Manager: David Zapanta

Callisto and the colophon are registered trademarks of Callisto Publishing LLC.

All rights reserved. No part of this book may be reproduced in any form or by any electronic or mechanical means including information storage and retrieval systems—except in the case of brief quotations embodied in critical articles or reviews—without permission in writing from its publisher, Sourcebooks LLC.

All brand names and product names used in this book are trademarks, registered trademarks, or trade names of their respective holders. Callisto Publishing is not associated with any product or vendor in this book.

Published by Callisto Publishing LLC C/O Sourcebooks LLC
P.O. Box 4410, Naperville, Illinois 60567-4410
(630) 961-3900
callistopublishing.com

Printed in the United States of America.

Emilene, this book is for you:
the life of the party, the giver of cuddles,
and the daughter God made for me.
I pray that you will always know, love,
and serve the Lord.

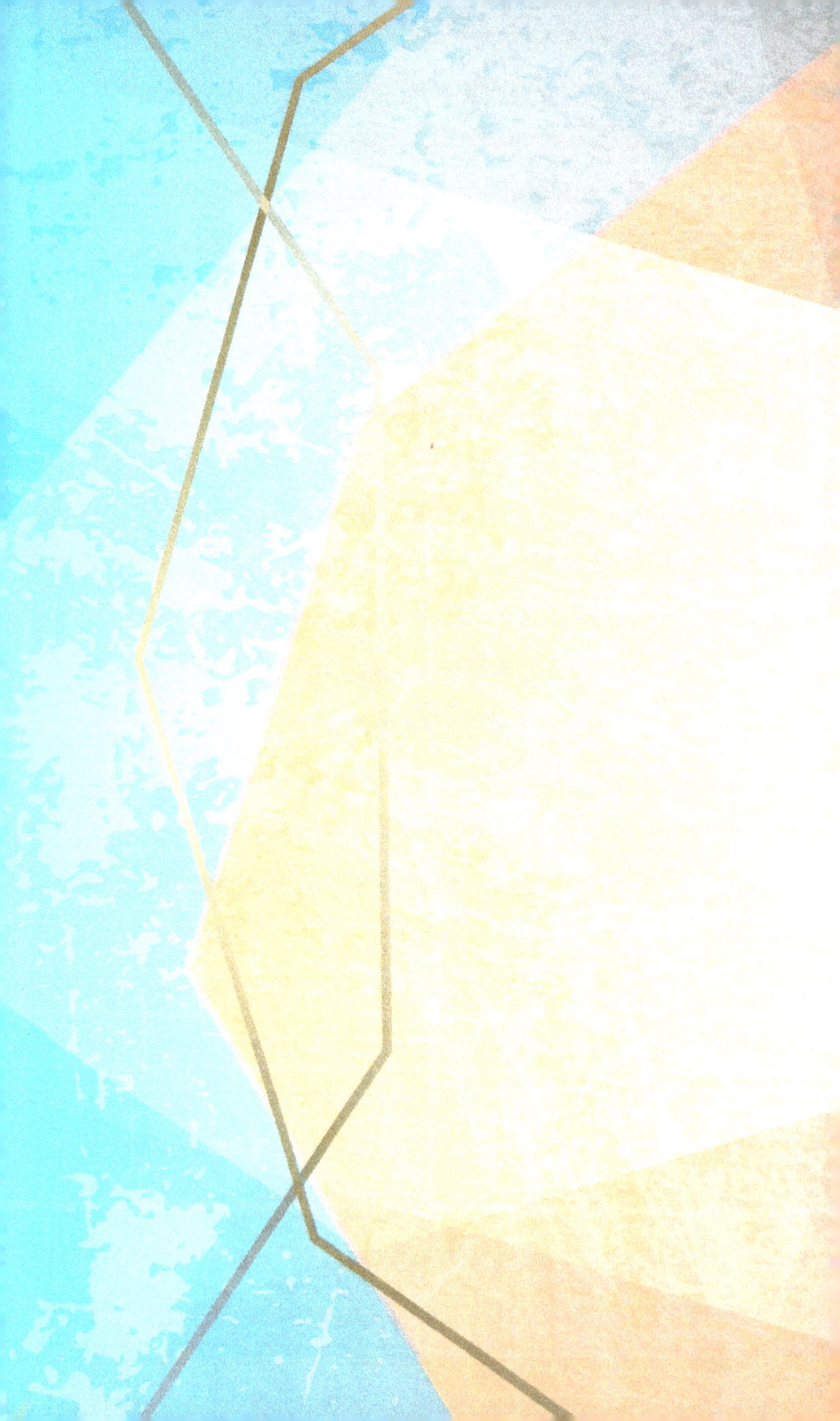

CONTENTS

Introduction xi
Day 1: Family of Faith 2
Day 2: Iron Sharpens Iron 4
Day 3: Raising Arrows 6
Day 4: Where Help Is Found 8
Day 5: Changing World, Same God 10
Day 6: Fearfully and Wonderfully Made 12
Day 7: Perfect Peace 14
Day 8: The Good Shepherd 16
Day 9: Words of Death or Life 18
Day 10: Perfect Peace 20
Day 11: Stay Strong 22
Day 12: Listening Well 24
Day 13: Persistent Prayer 26
Day 14: Strong in the Lord 28
Day 15: Mind What Matters 30
Day 16: Developing Self-Control 32
Day 17: The Secret to Contentment 34

Day 18: Pray Always 36

Day 19: Trusting and Growing 38

Day 20: A Generous Heart 40

Day 21: Endurance, Character, Hope 42

Day 22: Patience Is Tied to Love 44

Day 23: From Heavy to Light 46

Day 24: Temporary Home 48

Day 25: See What God Sees 50

Day 26: Worth > Worries 52

Day 27: The Helper Is Here 54

Day 28: Forgive Like Jesus 56

Day 29: A Gospel-Centered Life 58

Day 30: The Gift of Wisdom 60

Day 31: Give It Your All 62

Day 32: You Are His 64

Day 33: Doubts Are Welcome 66

Day 34: Know His Ways 68

Day 35: What Love Is and Isn't 70

Day 36: We Need Him 72

Day 37: True Beauty 74

Day 38: The Real Battleground 76

Day 39: The Joy in Trials 78

Day 40: Eternal Hope 80

Day 41: Creation's Sermon 82

Day 42: The Word of Life 84

Day 43: The Suffering Servant 86

Day 44: Stay Awake 88

Day 45: There's Always a Way Out 90

Day 46: Our Refuge, Our Strength,
Our Safety . . . Our God 92

Day 47: Put Off and Put On 94

Day 48: Imitators of God 96

Day 49: Deserve Is a Dirty Word 98

Day 50: God's Plans Are Always Better 100

Day 51: Truth Over Lies 102

Day 52: Approval That Matters 104

Day 53: The God Who Sees 106

Day 54: Suit Up 108

Day 55: Peace 110

Day 56: Give Your Fear to the Lord 112

Day 57: Using the Bad for the Good 114

Day 58: Every Good and Perfect Gift 116

Day 59: Worship as a Way of Life 118

Day 60: God of Hope 120

A Final Word 123

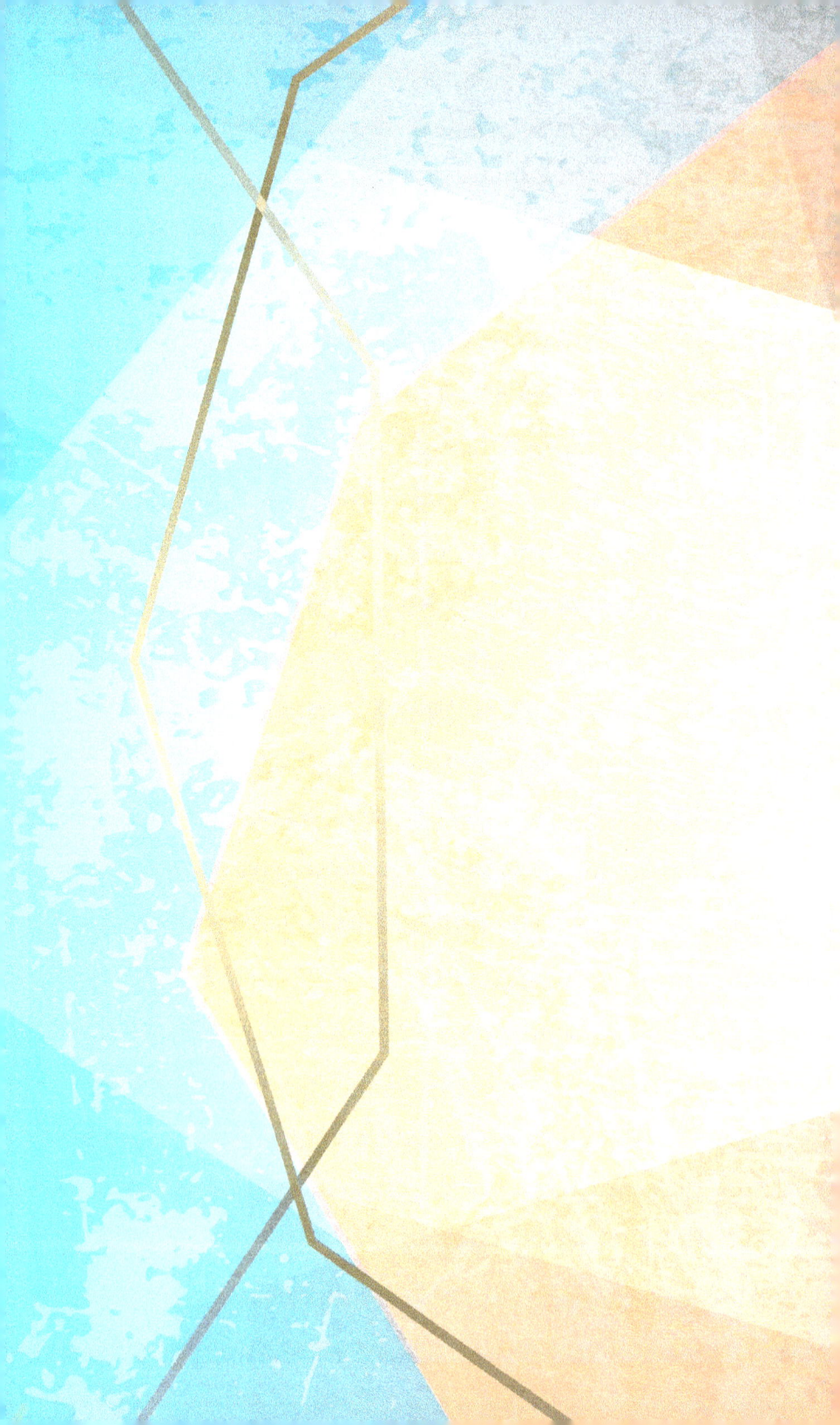

INTRODUCTION

I'm so glad you picked up this 60-day devotional. From one mom to another, I know that raising daughters can feel challenging and scary. I also know that raising girls is a privilege. It's exciting, fun, and an immense blessing.

I'm a mom, a wife, and a follower of Jesus. I was raised by a wonderful woman of God, who was also raised by a wonderful woman of God. Now I'm raising my own daughter, and I'm thankful to have been given such a great example by the women in my family. I'm also grateful that God is with me every step of the way. He's there for the good and the bad, when I have a great parenting moment and when I really screw up . . . which I do. The great news is that if He's there for me, He's there for you, too.

As moms, most of us start out unsure, and it's a feeling that can plague us throughout parenthood. I remember when we left the hospital with our first child, I had a sinking feeling that they shouldn't let me leave with him; I really had no clue what I was doing. I double-checked that car seat 100 times and sat in the back seat holding our baby's head while my husband drove home like we were traveling over a minefield. Does any of this sound remotely familiar to you?

Rest assured that being unsure is normal. But just because it's common doesn't mean we can't or shouldn't search for guidance and wisdom. In fact, we *should* search for those things, because we will find them when we look in the right places.

That's why I've written this devotional. The best place to find wisdom and guidance is God's Word. As a mom who loves the Lord and His Word, I want to encourage and equip other moms, too. Over the next 60 days, we'll learn from scripture so we can grow as mothers and build stronger relationships with our daughters. Together we will look honestly at the challenges facing our daughters in this world and think biblically about how best to prepare them.

This book is for all moms of daughters. Whether your daughter is a heartbeat that still lies inside you or is on the cusp of adulthood, it's always a good time to soak yourself in the truth and encouragement of scripture. If you've picked up this book, you know how important it is to seek guidance, wisdom, encouragement, and inspiration from the Word. This is important not only for your daughter's sake but for your own, too.

We live in an amazing time with so many wonderful Bible translations. For this book, I'll be quoting from the English Standard Version (ESV) unless otherwise noted, but whatever version you have is great. Which version you use isn't a consideration for this book. As Christian moms, we love Jesus and look to Him above all else. That is what we all have in common, and that is the perspective this devotional is built upon.

Now let's begin!

How to Use This 60-Day Devotional

Even though this devotional is created with your busy life in mind, I do recommend setting aside time each day to enjoy some quiet and read each day's devotion. I prefer mornings, before my feet hit the floor. Perhaps you prefer to linger over the day's devotion while you sip your morning coffee or in the evening after the kids are tucked in. Every life is different; you need to do what's best for you!

Regardless of how you approach this devotional, you'll discover that each time you open it up, you'll find a verse, a devotion, two reflection questions, an action of the day, and a guided prayer. The questions are to help you think more deeply, the action is so you can get practical, and the guided prayer is simply to help focus your heart and soul as you talk to God. Remember, a new routine can be challenging. Have patience with yourself as you begin this devotional. Just as God has shown us so much grace, reserve some grace for yourself, as well.

Enjoy God's Lesson

This devotional is not meant to add pressure to an already busy life. Think of it as breathing life into a heart that may be weary. This book is meant to inspire you, draw you close to God, and give you confidence and encouragement as you go about the incredibly important job of raising your daughter(s).

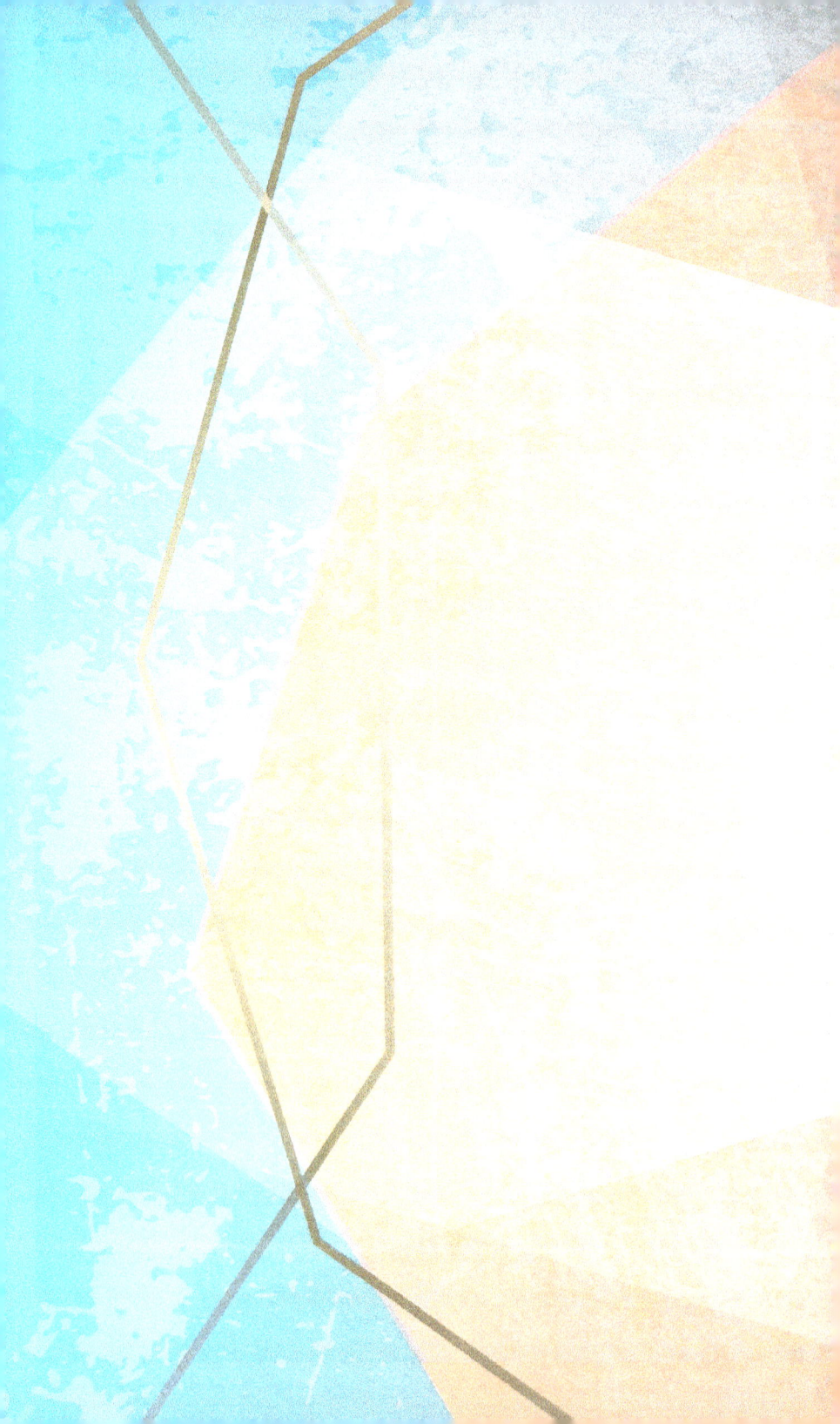

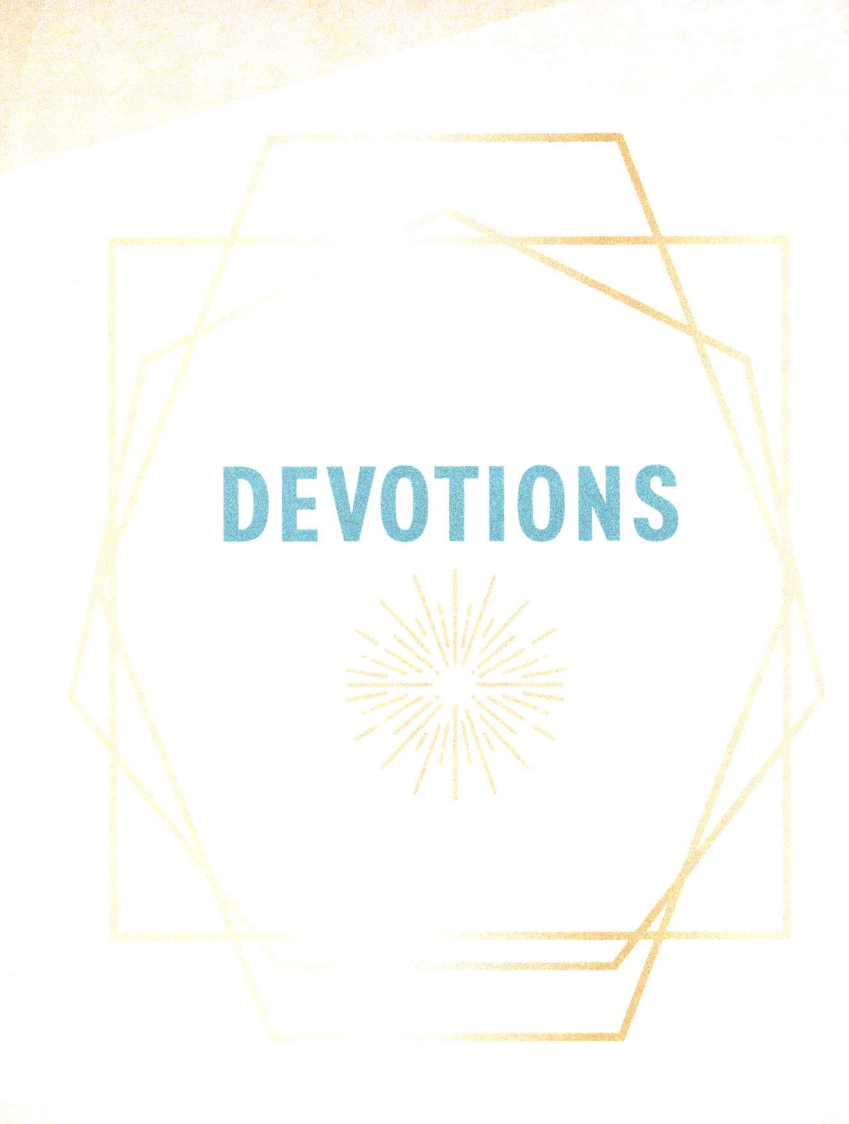

DAY 1
Family of Faith

I am reminded of your sincere faith, a faith that dwelt first in your grandmother Lois and your mother Eunice and now, I am sure, dwells in you as well.

2 TIMOTHY 1:5

In the introduction of this book, I spoke briefly about my mom and my grandma. I want you to get to know them a little better. My grandma's name is Hermina, and she's now 87 years old. She's a woman of deep faith, humility, and kindness. When I think of my grandma, I think of comfort and peace. I think of the quiet way she would read stories to me as a little girl. I think of the reverence in her voice when she reads the Bible. And I think of her writing. I could recognize her penmanship anywhere. I was blessed to receive a handwritten note of encouragement and prayer in every birthday card she gave me.

My mom's name is Marlene. She is strong, capable, giving, and present. When I think back on my childhood, I have no doubt in my mind that my mom was the person I trusted most and felt most comfortable around. Her prayers brought me through dark times, and her dependence on God in the midst of her busy life was so evident.

For both of those amazing women, God isn't just a piece of their lives that they've tucked away for Sundays. He is real, living, and in every moment. He isn't an occasion or a tradition; He is the reason for everything.

Just as Timothy (from today's scripture passage) had a strong example of godly women in his life, so do I. And so does your daughter. The gift of a godly mother is a prize worth more than gold. Our daughters listen to the words we say (well, sometimes), but more than that, they observe the lives we live. Be the godly example she needs.

In your home, don't make God an occasion or a tradition. Put Him front and center. Model what it looks like to live a life dependent on and inspired by the Lord. In doing so, and with prayer, you'll see your daughter draw closer to the Lord, as well.

LET'S REFLECT

- What woman in your life has been a godly example for you? What impact has the presence or absence of that person had on you?
- In your home, is God simply for Sundays, or is He for all the time? What are ways you model your faith for your daughter?

TAKE ACTION: Today, while you're cooking or hanging around the house, turn on some worship music. Sing along to it with your daughter. Engage her in your worship, and have fun together.

LET'S PRAY

God, I thank You that I know You. There is no greater privilege than to be Your child and to be trusted as a mother. I pray You will help me live a life of sincere faith and that my daughters will follow the same path. Amen.

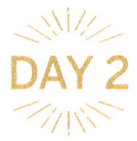

DAY 2

Iron Sharpens Iron

Iron sharpens iron, and one man sharpens another.

PROVERBS 27:17

I love to play tennis. Something about that ball popping off the racket is so satisfying. The thing is, though, I'm no superstar. I mean, I'm not terrible, but I'm not winning any awards, either. I know that for me to get better at it, I need to play with someone. Hitting a tennis ball against a wall by myself only gets me so far, and occasionally, it bounces off the wall and straight into my face. So, I play tennis with my husband. When I'm playing against him, I have to be stronger and faster. I also learn from watching him. I may not win much when I play against him, but he sharpens my skills.

    The same is true in motherhood. If we isolate ourselves and take the approach of "I don't need anyone," we won't stay sharp. In fact, we'll get dull really quickly. If you're finding that you're feeling dull, this doesn't mean you don't have the tools you need to be a great girl mom—you do! You just need someone beside you who can sharpen you and whom you can sharpen in return.

    God created us for community. He created us to support each other and to build each other up. He calls us to carry each other's burdens (Galatians 6:2). By surrounding yourself with a community of other women, you will be modeling for your daughter what it looks like to live in a healthy community where people are supported, challenged, and sharpened.

    You've lived enough life to know that there are going to be times in your daughter's life that are hard. You know she's going to encounter circumstances that are new and possibly frightening.

Show her that iron sharpens iron—and people sharpen people—so that she can be as strong and fortified as possible for whatever she may encounter in life.

LET'S REFLECT

- Do you lean more toward isolation or community? What impact has this had on your faith and your motherhood?
- Iron sharpens iron. Name one person (or more) in your life who could sharpen you as a mother, and consider how you can sharpen your daughter as well.

TAKE ACTION: Today, seek out wisdom from the person you identified as someone who may sharpen you. This may mean sitting down for coffee together, having a phone conversation, or sending a quick text. Let that person know you appreciate the role they have in your life.

LET'S PRAY

God, sometimes I'm tempted to try to do everything myself. I pray that You'll remind me that I need other people to help me grow as a woman, as a mother, and as Your child. Please put people in my daughters' lives who will sharpen them as well. Amen.

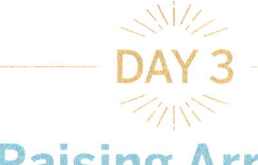

DAY 3

Raising Arrows

Behold, children are a heritage from the Lord, the fruit of the womb a reward. Like arrows in the hand of a warrior are the children of one's youth.

PSALM 127:3–4

When my son was eight, he got a fish named Dumbo. He was a nice fish who liked to swim around and put on a show. My son was very dedicated to feeding him and keeping his tank clean. He considered him a blessing and a responsibility. So when Dumbo died within a year, my son was devastated. He now has a new fish, named Bumbo. I know, the originality of the second name compared to the first is *truly* inspiring.

And as much as my son considered his fish a blessing, it makes me think about how much of a blessing my children are to me. It is a reward and a true gift that God has trusted us with our children. Each time we look into our children's eyes, we have the amazing ability to see the evidence of God's blessing.

Along with being a blessing, our kids are a huge responsibility. We do a lot of things in life, but our kids take the most consistent and attentive work. Raising them is not an eight-hour workday where you get to clock out when you've put in your time. It is nonstop, important, holy work.

You see, our children aren't really ours. Before they were born, they were the Lord's, and in the end, they're always His. We're just the ones whom He trusted here on Earth to bring them up to be *arrows*.

What do I mean by arrows? An arrow is carefully made, chosen by a warrior, aimed, and shot at a precise target. As moms raising girls, we're raising arrows. We get to diligently craft the arrow. We get to point it and let it fly in the direction it should go. Our goal is not just to raise "nice girls" but to raise strong women who choose to happily offer themselves as God's instruments here on Earth.

What a privilege.

LET'S REFLECT

- When you think about raising your daughter, what are your goals not only for her future, but for her character?
- Today's scripture reminds us of the blessing that our girls are, as well as the responsibility. With this in mind, are you being intentional in your moments with your daughter?

TAKE ACTION: Today, spend time chatting with your daughter about her future. Focus on what her character will be like when she's older. Get her perspective on the kind of woman she'd like to be, and help mold her into the arrow God intended her to be.

LET'S PRAY

I am humbled You chose me to be the mother of my daughters. They are Yours first, and it is my job to steward the beautiful gift You have given me. Give me the wisdom I need to raise arrows—to raise my daughters—for Your glory. Amen.

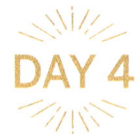

DAY 4

Where Help Is Found

I lift up my eyes to the hills. From where does my help come? My help comes from the Lord, who made heaven and earth.

PSALM 121:1–2

Before I had kids, I lived a very controlled life. I chose the "right" career for a stable life, I rose quickly in the professional ranks, I was overprepared for everything (to the point of anxiety), and I convinced myself that I could control anything that came my way.

But then one day, God stepped in. When I became pregnant with my first child, He showed me that I couldn't control everything. I couldn't control the state of my pregnancy, or how the birth went. I couldn't control the fact that my baby was born sick and stayed sick for years. I couldn't control the fact that my body and mind were spent, and I was diagnosed with an autoimmune disease when my baby was less than a year old.

I went from being a girl who didn't need or want help from anyone but herself to being a woman who realized I needed more help than I could give myself, and more help than any human could give me. I needed help from God.

Psalm 121 was one of my grandpa's favorite Bible verses. As a child I had it memorized. But it wasn't until I was a woman, at the end of the rope I had created for myself, that those words became real. That was when those words became alive. I was a mother by the time I realized that those words were the truth I was searching for all along.

I learned that there is nothing like motherhood to humble you quickly and permanently. As you're raising your daughter, you will undoubtedly need the support of a community around you. But more than that, you need to remember that help comes from the Lord, the maker of heaven and earth . . . and the maker of you.

LET'S REFLECT

- Are you someone who is willing to accept help from others? From the Lord?
- Can you think of a time in your life when God has reminded you that He is sovereign and you are not?

TAKE ACTION: Read Psalm 121 with your daughter, and begin memorizing it together. By committing it to memory now, your daughter will have that comforting scripture in her heart and mind when she needs it most.

LET'S PRAY

Thank You that You are sovereign and I am not. Forgive me when I try to wrestle control from You. Thank You for mercifully reminding me that You are where my help is ultimately found. I pray that my daughters would know this truth deep in their souls. Amen.

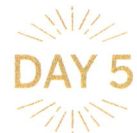

DAY 5

Changing World, Same God

Jesus Christ is the same yesterday and today and forever.

HEBREWS 13:8

The car. The airplane. The gun. The lightbulb. The telephone. Penicillin.

What do these things have in common? They were all inventions or discoveries that changed the course of this world. The other thing they all have in common is that they were invented or discovered long before you and I were born.

One thing that was invented in my lifetime is the iPhone. This invention changed the world once again. I remember the first time I saw an iPhone. My older brother had bought one, and we were sitting around the kitchen table together having coffee. He was showing me the phone, and I remember, clear as day, being completely floored when he flipped the phone and the image on the screen flipped at the same time. Sorcery. At least, that's how I felt at that moment.

Since 2011 (I was a somewhat late adopter), my iPhone has been a part of my everyday life. As with anything, there's good and bad that come along with it, but the bad has become increasingly obvious. Everyone is now carrying around a little computer in their pocket. Anyone can access pornography or any type of inappropriate, problematic content, whenever they want. Social media has become increasingly prevalent and divisive. We are wasting more time than ever before.

The world is changing rapidly, and it will continue to do so. Some changes will be good, and some changes will be bad. Whether the change is good or bad, it can be difficult for our daughters to navigate a changing world. It can leave them feeling unsure, insecure, and untethered.

This verse in Hebrews reminds us that though things change all around us, Jesus never does. He is our anchor in every storm and our glory in every victory. Remind your daughter of that fact every day.

LET'S REFLECT

- How does our constantly shifting culture make you feel as an adult?
- Have you observed your daughter reacting anxiously to any changes in the world?

TAKE ACTION: Write out today's Bible verse on a sticky note and post it in a prominent area where both you and your daughter will see it each day. Let it serve as a reminder of our anchor in a changing world.

LET'S PRAY

Thank You, Lord, for always remaining the same. Your faithfulness has been evident since the beginning of time. Whenever we feel uncertain in this changing world, we are reassured by who You were, are, and will always be. Amen.

DAY 6

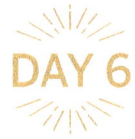

Fearfully and Wonderfully Made

I praise you, for I am fearfully and wonderfully made. Wonderful are your works; my soul knows it very well.

PSALM 139:14

The world we live in is not only noisy but saturated with images. A casual scroll on social media will reveal that there is a very different standard for men than there is for women. Women, in particular, are often portrayed online with careful filters, precise angles, and unrealistic expectations.

Women's bodies are often shown as if they are commodities, and the currency is likes, shares, and emojis. I've spoken with many teen girls who struggle with body image issues because of the media that saturates their daily lives and skews their reality. This leads many to feel unworthy, ugly, and unimportant when held up to the latest social media superstars. This is an assault on truth.

This reality can make us feel helpless in the midst of such a daunting and large issue. How are we to respond as women and mothers? How are we supposed to not only protect our daughters but equip them to see themselves as beautiful individuals made in the image of God, rather than just insignificant? Well, the answer lies in that very question.

Our job as mothers is to remind our daughters, without fail, that they are made on purpose, for a purpose, in the image of God: the Creator of the universe and everything in it. They weren't patched together unintentionally, without care or thought; they were *fearfully and wonderfully* made. They were made to be who they are by God, and all His works are wonderful.

Amid the noise and images battering this world, remind your daughter that she is beautiful. Not just because of how she looks, but because of who made her. May your constant reminders sink into her soul. When her soul recognizes her worth in light of her Creator, she will never question her beauty, her worthiness, or the fact that she is incomprehensibly and fully loved . . . just as she is.

LET'S REFLECT

- Do you ever feel fearful about bringing up a daughter in a world that portrays women in such an unrealistic way? What are some steps you can take to help her see her worth?
- You and your daughter were both created "fearfully and wonderfully." How does this make you feel?

TAKE ACTION: Today, tell your daughter some positive characteristics you see in her that have absolutely nothing to do with her appearance. Remind her that those characteristics are from God and that He intentionally gave her those qualities.

LET'S PRAY

Thank You for creating my daughters fearfully and wonderfully. Give me the wisdom to raise confident women in this culture that often tries to tear down rather than build up. You hold my daughters in Your hands. I pray that they will feel Your love and reassurance every day. Amen.

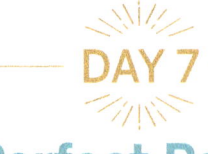

DAY 7

Perfect Peace

Do not be anxious about anything, but in everything by prayer and supplication with thanksgiving let your requests be made known to God. And the peace of God, which surpasses all understanding, will guard your hearts and your minds in Christ Jesus.

PHILIPPIANS 4:6–7

I was lying back in my zero-gravity chair, listening to the river run and the birds sing while reading a book. Total bliss. We were camping, and I was incredibly relaxed. Then I heard my daughter scream and cry. I rushed over, thinking she must have been stung by a bee, or much worse. When she was finally calm enough to speak, I found out she saw a spider. SAW a spider. It didn't bite her; it didn't touch her. She *saw* a spider while camping in the great outdoors (a truly shocking place to find a spider), and it was terrifying and devastating all rolled into one. Her anxiety about this horrible spider was understandable for a six year old. To her, that spider was big!

To me, as an adult, it seemed small and inconsequential. I may not run from spiders anymore, but there are things that scare me. I know some things scare you, too. I know this because we're moms. When we're raising future world-changers, it's easy to feel fearful. But God tells us a different story. A story that's important for us to remember, and a story that we must teach our daughters.

The story is this: We serve a God who listens to our prayers. He's not hands-off and aloof; He's in the weeds of this parenting gig with us. When we are persistent in prayer and continually remind ourselves of God's faithfulness, something truly amazing happens. We feel the peace of God, which surpasses all understanding and washes away every bit of anxiousness—be it from a spider or something much bigger.

This God-size peace will fill our hearts and minds and the hearts and minds of our daughters, too. Whether they're 2, 6, or 17, our daughters are just at the beginning. They've got beautiful lives in this big world stretching before them. Anxiety is real. It happens. So let's show our daughters where to find peace.

LET'S REFLECT

- Do you believe that God's peace can cast out worries? If you struggle with this, consider why.

- Have you noticed anxiety in yourself or your daughter? How does reading this passage of scripture make you feel?

TAKE ACTION: Today, put persistent prayer into practice, even if it feels hard to quiet your soul. Pray for your daughter's heart and mind. Pray that the peace of God would wash over her now and in her future. Model to your daughter what it looks like to have faith in the practice of prayer.

LET'S PRAY

Lord, You make no secret that life will be full of joy, challenge, beauty, and struggle, but Your Word reveals the way to peace. Wash my daughters and myself with peace, today and every day. May we never forget this perfect peace is a gift from You. Amen.

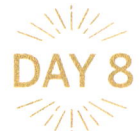

DAY 8

The Good Shepherd

The thief comes only to steal and kill and destroy. I came that they may have life and have it abundantly. I am the good shepherd. The good shepherd lays down his life for the sheep.

JOHN 10:10–11

Jesus calls Himself the good shepherd in this passage. In today's world this may not seem that significant, but shepherds were a big part of Israel's culture; even King David was a shepherd.

When reading this verse and the verses surrounding it, imagine a flock of sheep peacefully grazing. Lambs skipping and running, sheep chewing lazily, and the occasional bleat as the sheep communicate among themselves. Then suddenly, the peace is shattered when a mountain lion jumps over the fence and starts ravaging the sheep. Calm turns to chaos in an instant.

Now imagine that same peaceful scene we started with, happy lambs and content sheep. This time the shepherd steps into the pasture through the gate. He calls out to the sheep, and they run toward him, knowing that he is their safety and sustenance. They run toward him because they know that he would fight for them, even lay down his life for them.

In today's passage, Jesus casts himself as the good shepherd and the people as the sheep. The shepherd is the only one who would enter through the gate. All others enter by some other way, and they mean the sheep harm. Jesus uses this story to tell us that as a good shepherd cares for his sheep, so He cares for us.

We don't live in a perfect world. There are going to be people and circumstances that will try to steal and destroy the hearts and souls of our daughters. The answer for this is to teach them the voice of their shepherd. When they know His voice, they will run toward Him and away from the people or things that seek to harm them. When they know His voice, they will seek refuge in Him. And when they understand that He has laid down His life for them already, they will cling to Him in any circumstance.

LET'S REFLECT

- What do you think God is wanting you to take away from today's reading?
- In order to help your daughter recognize the Lord's voice, you have to recognize it as well. What are ways you can grow in closeness to the Lord?

TAKE ACTION: To help your daughter get to know Jesus, start reading through one of the gospels (Matthew, Mark, Luke, or John) together. You don't have to do a ton of reading every day. Even just a few verses each day will help your daughter get to know the Good Shepherd.

LET'S PRAY

God, I thank You for Your love and protection. Thank You for laying down Your life so that we could experience life abundantly. I pray that You will come alongside me as I train up my daughters to know You. I pray that as they grow, they will know You, love You, and serve You. Amen.

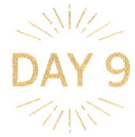

DAY 9

Words of Death or Life

*Death and life are in the power of the tongue,
and those who love it will eat its fruits.*

PROVERBS 18:21

It's incredibly important that as mothers raising daughters, we impart to our daughters the power of the words they say. To raise strong, confident, kind women, we need to teach them that words are not weak and listless but firm and influential, a unique and powerful way to connect. The way we use them, though, can bring darkness or light, death or life.

I searched for a scientific study that would tell us how many words a woman speaks in a day, but surprise, each study conflicted with the others. What we do know, though, is that we speak *thousands* of words per day. What a beautiful thing it would be for our daughters to not only speak but hear thousands of words each day that are filled with life and light.

As moms, we need to be thoughtful with our words. We need to choose self-control rather than outbursts, and we need to remember that not everything we think and feel has to be voiced immediately. As we lean into the Lord each day and choose to conform to Him rather than the world, He tells us that He will renew our minds. In doing this, we will be able to test and "discern what is the will of God, what is good and acceptable and perfect" (Romans 12:2).

It should always be our goal to lead by example and to commit our daughters to prayer. Showing ourselves grace is a perfect example. James 3:2 says, "If anyone does not stumble in what he says, he is a perfect man." We know none of us is perfect . . . this is why we need Jesus. We will make mistakes and say things we wish we hadn't. But then we get to lead by example again and show our daughters humility when we apologize.

Death and life are in the power of the tongue. Speak life with yours.

LET'S REFLECT

- As you were reading, what in particular stood out to you? Why?
- Reflect on a time when someone spoke words to you that brought light, and a time when words were spoken to you that brought darkness. How did each instance make you feel, and how can you learn from each and apply that learning to your motherhood?

TAKE ACTION: Today, speak words of encouragement and affirmation to each person you encounter. Especially your daughter! So often we think people know what we admire about them, but they may not. Be a blessing with your words today.

LET'S PRAY

God, I thank You for the beautiful gift of language. I thank You that I get to communicate and connect with people in such a unique way. I recognize that this blessing comes with responsibility, and I pray that You will help me use my words wisely. Please help me lead by example so that my daughters will see the beauty in speaking words of life instead of death. Amen.

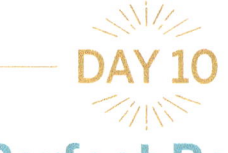

DAY 10

Perfect Peace

You keep him in perfect peace whose mind is stayed on you, because he trusts in you.

ISAIAH 26:3

On one hot sunny Sunday this past spring, I found myself sitting in the waiting area of an emergency room with my grandma. The ER was filled with people. Some were clutching a bag to their mouths, some were inebriated, some were kids with broken bones, and many were there with COVID-19.

My grandma hadn't been feeling well and had been having some unexplained symptoms. There was a question mark over what was causing her to feel unwell, and there was a laundry list of possibilities. She was uncomfortable, she was sick, but she wasn't anxious.

As we sat together, she told me that she finds great comfort in Isaiah 26:3. That verse is only a few words long, but it tells us a lot about God and a lot about what it's like to be someone who trusts in God. The brief words of that verse remind us that God is faithful. He's not just faithful because He says He is; He has the history to back it up.

Keeping our minds "stayed" on Him means that we recall His faithfulness over the years; we remember what He has done, not only for us but since the beginning of time. He provided a lamb for Abraham to sacrifice in place of Isaac. He took the sin of Joseph's brothers and turned it into opportunity. He provided manna in the desert. He provided His Son to atone for our sins.

Those are just a few of the many examples of God's faithfulness. In the biblical examples I gave, all of those people were going through a hard time. God didn't make everything "easy," but He provided what His people needed. In the same way, God doesn't promise that life will be easy for you. He doesn't promise that motherhood will be without challenges. But He does promise peace to the heart that is fixed on Him.

LET'S REFLECT

- What jumped out at you from today's reading? What does God want you to hear?
- When you consider peace, do you expect it will only come when everything is going well? How can you experience peace in the midst of challenges?

TAKE ACTION: It's so important for your daughter to know true peace. If you sense anxiety or worry in your daughter today, remind her of God's care for her in the past, and remind her that He will care for her the same way in the present and the future.

LET'S PRAY

God, I thank You for Your faithfulness, and I thank You for Your Word. Through it, You have provided a way for me to be constantly reminded of Your faithfulness. I pray that my daughters will see your faithfulness as well, and that they will be filled with Your perfect peace as they rest in the knowledge of Your sovereignty. Amen.

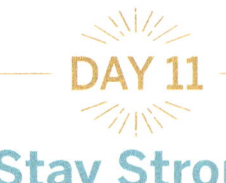

DAY 11

Stay Strong

And let us not grow weary of doing good, for in due season we will reap, if we do not give up.

GALATIANS 6:9

Like all good stories, this one starts with me scrubbing a toilet. Just kidding. That's not where all good stories start, but this one does start with me cleaning a toilet while crying my eyes out.

    At this time, my three kids were aged five and under, and I was working, dealing with my child's food allergies, and maintaining a somewhat tidy home. My kids had been filled with energy all day (both positive and negative), and I was done with playing referee and first-aid attendant. I had just put the kids to bed, and as I picked up that toilet brush, I couldn't help but let the tears fall. I was tapped out and exhausted.

    I felt bad for being frustrated with my kids. I felt like I had been a terrible example to them all day. After the toilet was clean, I went upstairs to apologize to my oldest. As I walked back into the bedroom he picked up his Etch-a-Sketch and said, "Look, Mommy!" He had drawn a beautiful picture of a cross on a hill with two crosses in the background.

    That simple picture was a beautiful reminder of God's grace. I had become weary of my life and all my responsibilities. But God didn't discard me in frustration when I began to falter. Instead, He used my child to remind me of why I do what I do every day. I don't do it so that I can feel good about myself. I don't do it so that my kids will be "successful" someday. And I don't do it to win any "mom" awards.

Just like you, I do the hard work of parenting every day because I want my kids to see the cross. There is nothing more important for our girls than for them to see Jesus and be transformed by Him. On one of my roughest days, God showed me what I needed to see. He showed me that my children see the cross. They see Jesus. And I will not grow weary or give up, because the reward the Lord offers is so great.

LET'S REFLECT

- In reading this today, could you identify with the feelings that were described? In what way?
- As you raise your daughter, what causes you to feel weary?

TAKE ACTION: Today, spend a couple of extra minutes praying that God would fortify you in your motherhood and remind you of the meaningful and eternal reasons for the important work you're doing as you raise your daughter.

LET'S PRAY

God, I thank You that You are a God of beautiful promises and faithful reminders. Thank You for the reminder today that You see me in the midst of this hard and holy work of parenting my daughters. I pray that You would strengthen me as I continue this important work. Amen.

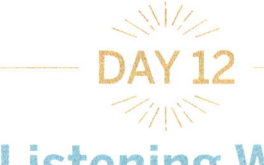

DAY 12
Listening Well

Know this, my beloved brothers: let every person be quick to hear, slow to speak, slow to anger.

JAMES 1:19

My daughter loves to color. She doesn't care whether she's coloring on paper, cardboard, carpet, or walls. I thought that was something that would only plague us throughout the toddler years, but no. She doesn't give up easily.

If you were to walk through our house, you would see evidence on almost every wall of her artwork. The stuff from her early years is mostly cleaned off, but as the years wore on, I got tired of scrubbing. And try as she might, she doesn't quite have the strength to get crayon or ink off walls.

She's six now, and her last work of art was just a couple of months ago. It was on our walls, and it was her name, written in huge letters up the stairs. When I saw what she had done, I guarantee you that I wasn't in the mood to be quick to hear, slow to speak, or slow to anger. In fact, it was the complete opposite. In the big picture, writing on walls and my reaction to it might seem small. But for her, these are big things! This is her six-year-old life, and watching the way I react is her training ground for how to respond when things happen to her.

What would happen if instead of being quick to chastise we are quick to hear? Whether we're speaking with our kids, our spouse, our coworkers, or a person with different political opinions, if we choose to really listen, we might hear something profound and beautiful, or something that awakens our understanding. If we choose to be patient rather than angry, we can build a bridge rather than burn one down.

Further on in that chapter of James, we read, "Receive with meekness the implanted word, which is able to save your souls" (James 1:21). The word "meekness" is defined in the Merriam-Webster Online Dictionary as "a mild, moderate, humble, or submissive quality." My take is that in order to be slow to speak, slow to anger, and quick to hear, we need to be humble. As mothers, we need to admit that we need the Lord and His Word implanted in us. We need His Word to change and shape us daily into the kind of people and mothers who truly are quick to hear, slow to speak, and slow to anger.

LET'S REFLECT

- Would you describe yourself as humble and meek? Whether you said yes or no, what personality characteristics make you think that?

- Have you ever experienced the kindness of someone who was quick to hear you rather than quick to speak or get angry?

TAKE ACTION: Pay attention to your conversations with your daughter today. Are you quick to hear or to speak? Take note of how the dynamics of your relationship and conversation shift when you actively and truly listen.

LET'S PRAY

Thank You for being a God who has such incredible mercy on Your children. Thank You for truly hearing me and relenting from Your anger and offering forgiveness. I pray that You would equip me to grow in that same character, and that as I do, my relationships with my daughters would be enriched. Amen.

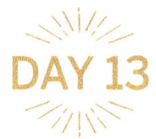

DAY 13
Persistent Prayer

And there was a widow in that city who kept coming to him and saying, "Give me justice against my adversary." For a while he refused, but afterward he said to himself, "Though I neither fear God nor respect man, yet because this widow keeps bothering me, I will give her justice, so that she will not beat me down by her continual coming."

LUKE 18:3–5

Today's passage is taken from Luke 18, and it is part of the Parable of the Persistent Widow. Grab your Bible and read the whole thing; it's a short eight verses. When you're done reading, you'll see that Jesus isn't talking to the people about how to be so annoying that you'll get what you want. He's using this parable to show us what God desires of us. As in all His parables, He's using a relatable story to make a deeper point.

The judge in this story is, by his own definition, not a great guy. He readily admits that he has no fear of God and no respect for people. All he cares about is that this widow is stealing his peace. He wants her to leave him alone.

So why would Jesus use this less-than-kind judge in a parable? He does this because He's trying to illustrate that even this *unrighteous judge* is willing to give justice when it's asked for persistently. How much *more willingly* will our loving Father give to those of us who are persistent in prayer?

Motherhood should come with a warning: **Do not attempt without prayer.** We are responsible for shaping and molding our children. We are charged with teaching them about God and life. Raising daughters is the kind of job that requires persistent prayer. We need to be knocking relentlessly on the door of heaven, asking for God's protection and provision over our girls. We need to become like the persistent widow. God will listen and act. And not because we're driving Him crazy, but because He loves us and delights in our prayers.

LET'S REFLECT

- What can you learn from the persistent widow?
- How does it make you feel that God wants to hear your prayers?

TAKE ACTION: Time to take a cue from the persistent widow. Today, pray for your daughter. Pray that she will know God, love God, and serve God. Pray for her protection and provision. Make a habit of this prayer.

LET'S PRAY

Thank You for loving me enough to request my prayers. Thank You for Your Word, which encourages my prayers. I pray that You will make me bold like the persistent widow. Please watch over my daughters, and draw them close to You. This is my daily plea. Amen.

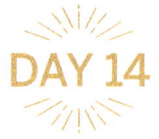

DAY 14

Strong in the Lord

"Have I not commanded you? Be strong and courageous. Do not be frightened, and do not be dismayed, for the Lord your God is with you wherever you go."

JOSHUA 1:9

I love this Bible verse so much, because it feels like we're being given a commission when we read it. In reality, God *was* giving Joshua a commission with these words. Moses had died, and God was setting Joshua over the people of Israel. In Joshua 1:1–9, God commands him to be strong and courageous three times.

When I think of sending my daughter out into the world, I want her to accept this charge and be strong and courageous. I don't believe she is ever too young to learn strength and courage. She may not be leading a nation through the desert and to the promised land, but she will be living a life of purpose and importance.

A couple of years ago, I was dealing with some of my own worries about my kids going out into the world. They were shy and were often the ones getting pushed to the back of the line because they weren't willing to fight for position. True, they were only in line to go down the slide, but it hurt my heart to think of them out there getting shoved around.

I decided to get this Bible verse from Joshua printed on a wooden sign with a map of the world. I stuck it right by our mudroom door so that every time our family came or went from the house, wherever in the world we were going, we would have a reminder that the Lord was with us. That daily reminder is a key part of helping our kids remember that with the Lord by their side, they do not need to fear.

Our daughters will encounter many challenges in life. Like my kids' challenges, maybe theirs will start at the park while they're waiting in line for the slide. Chances are, their challenges won't be anything like the ones Joshua was facing. But they will experience fear.

Fear is a normal emotion, and it's part of life. Just looking at an encouraging Bible verse each day won't be enough to hold fear at bay. But when we allow the Word and prayer to become an active part of our daily lives, it will begin to transform us and our daughters into women who are strong and courageous, because we have the Lord.

LET'S REFLECT

- Do you recognize the importance of equipping your daughter with strength and courage? Have you had conversations with her about this?
- What are some ways you can remind your daughter that the Lord is with her? What are some ways you can help her deal with fear in a healthy way?

TAKE ACTION: Today, plan a fun activity that will push you and your daughter out of your comfort zones. If she likes to read, try going on a hike. If she's into sports, try spending some time baking together in the kitchen. Use this as an opportunity to remind her that God is always with her, even when she feels fear.

LET'S PRAY

I thank You that I can look throughout the Bible and see countless examples of Your faithfulness. Each one reminds me that I don't need to fear and that I can be strong. Help me teach my daughters the same thing. May they be bold in life because You are beside them. Amen.

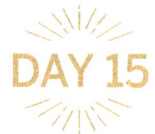

DAY 15

Mind What Matters

And he said to them, "You are those who justify yourselves before men, but God knows your hearts. For what is exalted among men is an abomination in the sight of God."

LUKE 16:15

Just before Jesus said this to a group of Pharisees, He had been telling a parable about a dishonest manager. The parable ended with Jesus saying, "No servant can serve two masters, for either he will hate the one and love the other, or he will be devoted to the one and despise the other. You cannot serve God and money" (Luke 16:13).

When the Pharisees heard Jesus say this, they began to make fun of Him. But Jesus could see right through them. He knew that the Pharisees loved money. They loved the honor that they received because of their position. They valued things that people valued. But when you're standing in front of the Son of God, he cuts through the nonsense and straight to the truth.

We live in a world that is cluttered with materialism. Girls are told what to wear, how to look, what to buy, what to think, and what to say. None of those things, though, are based on what God says matters. All of those things are based on what the world says matters.

When we fall prey to the demands of the world ourselves, we leave a wide door for our daughters to follow the same path. But God knows our hearts. Are we seeking to impress our fellow humans? Or are we seeking to please the Lord? Do we want our girls to go through life feverishly trying to stay relevant? Or do we want them to walk through life with the deep peace of knowing that the Lord loves a heart that is fully committed to what He says matters . . . regardless of the opinions of those around them?

You cannot serve two masters. Choose to serve the one who loved you so much that He chose to become human, suffer and die, then defeat death to promise you life.

LET'S REFLECT

- What from today's reading resonated with you the most? Have you been tempted to serve two masters?
- What are some steps you can take to start showing your daughter that what the world values is not what God values?

TAKE ACTION: Take some time today to assess what you prioritize in life. Consider whether it is in line with what the Lord says matters.

LET'S PRAY

Lord, I pray that as I raise my daughters in this world, You would give me the wisdom I need to put You ahead of earthly things. Give me the wisdom to model a life built on You rather than on temporary approval from others here on Earth. Thank You for Your patience as I grow to be more like You each day. Amen.

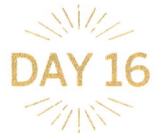

DAY 16

Developing Self-Control

Every athlete exercises self-control in all things. They do it to receive a perishable wreath, but we an imperishable. So I do not run aimlessly; I do not box as one beating the air. But I discipline my body and keep it under control, lest after preaching to others I myself should be disqualified.

1 CORINTHIANS 9:25–27

No one is born "good" at self-control. My mind flashes to a memory of my daughter around age three, stealing the peanut butter jar and hiding with it. When I found her, she was sticking her hand into the jar and eating the peanut butter like Winnie the Pooh would eat honey.

It's like kids have no self-control at all. I mean, have you seen how they pick their noses? But just because our kids start with little to no self-control doesn't mean they should stay that way. It's our job as mothers to help them grow in this important and biblical skill.

The instances above are really basic examples of losing self-control. But as tiny humans, kids don't have much self-control to lose, because they haven't had much time to develop it in their short existence. The development of self-discipline takes place in two complementary ways.

The first way we develop self-discipline is through the work of the Holy Spirit. 2 Timothy 1:6–7 says, "For this reason I remind you to fan into flame the gift of God, which is in you through the laying on of my hands, for God gave us a spirit not of fear but of power and love and self-control." These Bible verses make it clear that self-control is a gift of the Spirit. When we come to know Jesus, our self-control is primed to grow because of the work He will do in us.

Because we are given this gift, it is our job to steward it and grow it. That's where we run into the *second* way we grow in self-control: action. Action is where we take that gift of the Spirit and apply it. So whether our girls really are training as future Olympians or they're just training as future women and leaders, we need to help give them the tools and skills they need, including self-control.

LET'S REFLECT

- In general, do you think self-control is prized or minimized in our culture?
- Do you struggle with self-control? Have you seen your daughter struggle with self-control? In what areas?

TAKE ACTION: For today's action, I want to share some practical ways you can help your daughter grow in self-control. Pick one of these to work on today:

- Encourage her to spend time with God.
- Explain to her that we can't control everything, but we do have a lot of control over many of our choices.
- Help her develop and learn the value of boundaries.
- Remind her that, just as being an athlete of Olympic caliber doesn't just "happen," neither does perfect self-control. It's something we work at every day.

LET'S PRAY

We live in a world with fast access to so many things. I pray that You would help me balance thankfulness for the provisions You've given me with self-control. Help me model self-control well for my daughters so that they can grow into strong and grounded people. Amen.

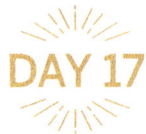

DAY 17

The Secret to Contentment

I know how to be brought low, and I know how to abound. In any and every circumstance, I have learned the secret of facing plenty and hunger, abundance and need. I can do all things through him who strengthens me.

PHILIPPIANS 4:12–13

Paul wrote these verses while he was in a jail cell. It was a Roman jail, in the time before electricity. Paul found himself in prison during days of severe oppression, racism, and division. He was a man who had faced incredible challenges and hardship. Yet we don't find him face down in anguish because life hasn't gone according to his plans. Instead, we find him rejoicing.

If you read all the way through Philippians, you may even find it to be one of the most joyful books in the Bible. The word "rejoice" is used abundantly. Why would Paul write in such a heartening tone when he is in the middle of being brought so low? And why, when we often find ourselves with so much, do we find ourselves unhappy?

Paul says that he found the secret to being content. We all like to know a secret . . . do you know what his secret was? The secret was that he didn't find contentment based on *circumstances*. His contentment came from the gospel. His contentment came from the message and the truth of Jesus Christ.

And that is where our contentment should be found as well. Our daughters are watching us through all of life's ups and downs. They are watching as the waves rock us back and forth, and they are seeing where we put our hope. I know for sure that storms will come and that the waves are going to rock our daughters one day.

RAISING GIRLS: DEVOTIONAL FOR MOM

Their choice will be to either focus on the storm or focus on the Savior. Let's show them how to choose Jesus over the storm.

LET'S REFLECT

- What jumped out at you from today's reading?
- Trusting God means putting your hope in something bigger than the world. Does this fill you with confidence or trepidation? Why?

TAKE ACTION: Today, whether you're tired or full of energy, sad or happy, winning or losing, focus on the beauty that God has placed around you and the good that He has done for you. Make a list of five things you're thankful for today.

LET'S PRAY

God, You are so good. Though the hardships of this world will try to cloud my faith, I pray that I will always cling to You. May You remind me constantly that my contentment isn't circumstantial but spiritual. I pray that You will draw my daughters close to You, that You will be their solid place to stand and the source of their joy. Amen.

DAY 18

Pray Always

Rejoice always, pray without ceasing, give thanks in all circumstances; for this is the will of God in Christ Jesus for you.

1 THESSALONIANS 5:16–18

Three short verses, so much goodness. It's interesting to me that "pray without ceasing" is a verse all on its own. Just three little words. Pray without ceasing. That's a lot of praying.

Prayer is an area that I'm trying to grow in. I've had times in my life when prayer was as natural as breathing and other times when it seemed forced, stale, and ineffective. It's in those times, though, that we need to press in even harder to prayer.

Prayer is one of the most important things we as mothers can do for our daughters. God wants us petitioning Him daily on behalf of our daughters . . . because they're His daughters, too! Today's Bible verse even says that this consistent prayer is actually "the will of God in Christ Jesus for you." That's a big deal. That tells us that if we aren't praying, we are going against the will of God.

This sentiment is reinforced in the Old Testament. In 1 Samuel, we find Israel about to have their first king, Saul. Samuel, a prophet, is talking to the people and reminding them of their sins. Then, in 1 Samuel 12:23, Samuel says, "Moreover, as for me, far be it from me that I should sin against the Lord by ceasing to pray for you, and I will instruct you in the good and the right way."

In that verse and the surrounding passage, we may be reading what a prophet was saying to the nation of Israel, but it reminds me of motherhood. Our daughters are going to do things that we don't understand. They're going to frustrate us and leave us feeling concerned. But just like Samuel, we have a responsibility to teach our daughters and to continually pray for them. To fail to do that would be a sin.

Do not cease to pray for your daughter, and do not cease to instruct her in the good and right way. It is your duty.

LET'S REFLECT

- Is prayer an area you struggle in? If so, why do you think this might be?
- Do you find it harder or easier to pray for your daughter when she has done something wrong? Why do you think this is?

TAKE ACTION: Today, pray for your daughter. You will be led in a short guided prayer at the end of today's devotion, but use it as a springboard to propel you deeper into prayer for your daughter.

LET'S PRAY

God, I thank You for my daughters. I thank You for trusting me to be their mother. I pray that You would equip me with the wisdom and strength I need to mother them well. I pray that You will draw them to you. As they grow, may they know You, love You, and serve You. I ask this in the name of Jesus. Amen.

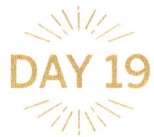

DAY 19

Trusting and Growing

I thank him who has given me strength, Christ Jesus our Lord, because he judged me faithful, appointing me to his service.

1 TIMOTHY 1:12

I wish I could sit here and tell you that I'm a perfect mom, but I can't. One area that I really need to grow in is letting my kids help with things. I'd much rather clean the house by myself to guarantee that it will be done well and quickly. I also don't like to relinquish the keys to the kitchen . . . I do not like to hand over the spatula. It's not because I love cooking. Quite the opposite, in fact. I loathe cooking and baking and want it done ASAP. If I have to take the time to teach my kids, it will just take longer and likely be messier.

When I don't allow them to help, though, it has an impact on them. They feel that I don't trust them or want them around. This isn't true, but I can understand why they'd see it that way. The way I do things is very different from the way God does things.

In this passage from 1 Timothy, Paul is writing about how thankful he is that Christ strengthened him. He goes on to describe how much he sinned and that it is only by God's grace and mercy that he was empowered to do the work of the kingdom. Paul, like you and me, is part of the body of Christ.

I admit that I like to hold responsibilities close to myself. Contrast that with how the Lord actually makes us part of His *body*. He doesn't keep us at a distance so that things are efficient and tidy; He makes us part of Himself to empower us to do more. This is a beautiful picture of how we should be leading our kids, and it's a truth that speaks to my mama heart.

LET'S REFLECT

- When you consider being part of the body of Christ, have you ever considered that as Christ empowering you?
- Do you empower your daughter, both in daily tasks and in her faith? If not, what can you do differently?

TAKE ACTION: Today, let your daughter help you with something you'd usually keep to yourself. Encourage her in her work.

LET'S PRAY

God, I pray that You would make me more like You. Instead of holding tight to responsibility and power, I pray that You would help me instead empower others, especially my daughters. Amen.

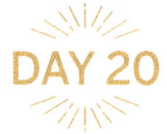

DAY 20

A Generous Heart

Sell your possessions, and give to the needy. Provide yourselves with moneybags that do not grow old, with a treasure in the heavens that does not fail, where no thief approaches and no moth destroys. For where your treasure is, there will your heart be also.

LUKE 12:33–34

This is a devotional for moms of daughters, but today, I'm going to use an example about my sons. This morning, I was getting ready to bring them to camp. They had a list of things they needed, and the last things they needed to grab before we got in the car were a hat and shoes. Well, this is when the problem started.

Despite the fact that we have more than a couple of hats, both boys wanted to wear the same one. There were disagreements over who had it first, whom it really belonged to, and so on. As I said, they may be boys, but I would be really surprised if you haven't been in a similar situation with your daughter.

My boys had decided that one particular hat was their treasure for the day, and they were willing to drag each other through the mud for it. At the time, neither was willing to be generous and offer the hat to his brother. In that moment, where their treasure was, so were their hearts.

Generosity is right near the core of Christianity. After all, we serve a God who was generous enough to offer His Son for our sins. We serve a Lord who was willing to leave His throne in heaven to come to the dirt of the earth and face death for us. It doesn't get more generous than that. Because generosity has been modeled on such a scale for us, we must model it and teach it to our daughters as well.

If we back up today's scripture passage to verse 32, it says, "Fear not, little flock, for it is your Father's good pleasure to give you the kingdom." It is His *pleasure* to give us the kingdom. What a gift! He doesn't give begrudgingly or under duress; He gives with pleasure. Let's do the same by giving generously to our daughters and to others and by giving our daughters the opportunity to give generously of their time, talents, and resources, as well. It's never too early to start being generous.

LET'S REFLECT

- What does it mean to you that God has been so generous to you?
- Can you think of a time when someone was really generous to you? How did that feel?

TAKE ACTION: Today, do something to model generosity for your daughter. Take her out for ice cream, spend time giving each other manicures, or go for a coffee date. In doing this, you'll model generosity and reap the bonus benefit of spending precious moments with your daughter.

LET'S PRAY

Lord, You have been so good to me. It is easy to want and want some more, but I pray that instead, You will help me give and then give some more. I pray that You would make me a joyful giver—not someone who gives because they have to, but someone who gives because I'm thankful. I pray the same for my daughters. Amen.

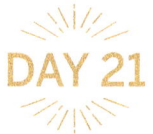

DAY 21

Endurance, Character, Hope

Not only that, but we rejoice in our sufferings, knowing that suffering produces endurance, and endurance produces character, and character produces hope, and hope does not put us to shame, because God's love has been poured into our hearts through the Holy Spirit who has been given to us.

ROMANS 5:3–5

Something I say often is that I wouldn't want to know who I would be if I hadn't gone through hard things in life. I didn't face any real challenges until I had kids, they got sick, and I got sick. Prior to this, I was uptight, controlling, and just fearful; I was fearful of failure, opinions, and judgment. If I hadn't had challenges in my life, I would have continued down a selfish and destructive path.

Having gone through some hard things, though, I can confidently say that sufferings are something we can rejoice in. This doesn't mean that they're fun. It doesn't mean that I excitedly anticipate the day when my own daughter faces challenges and opposition . . . but it does mean that I can have a God-given perspective and anticipate the refinement that is surely going to come from trials.

This passage says that suffering produces endurance, endurance produces character, and character produces hope. Go through that bit by bit, and see whether you can dispute it. Suffering does produce endurance, because you have no choice but to keep going when things are crumbling. The clock still moves, your heart still beats, and your lungs still draw breath. Suffering produces endurance.

Endurance produces character. This is true because when you persist and keep on through difficulty, you will have no choice but to grow stronger. Just as weight training causes muscles to break down, challenge is a struggle for our character. But then our muscles are repaired and grow stronger . . . just as our character does when faced with adversity.

Character produces hope. Yes. Because when you've been through the fire and find the flame hasn't consumed you (Isaiah 43:2), hope grows.

Maybe you're facing difficulty right now. Maybe your daughter is. Believe and know that no suffering is in vain. It produces endurance, character, hope, and the realization that Christ's love is in you and that the Holy Spirit is strengthening you daily.

LET'S REFLECT

- Have you experienced this progression from suffering to endurance to character building to hope in your own life? How did it change you?

- Our instinct as mothers is often to shield our daughters from all pain and disappointment. How has today's Bible passage shifted this for you?

TAKE ACTION: Share a story with your daughter today of a hard time you went through in your life. Highlight the work that God did in you throughout that experience.

LET'S PRAY

God, I thank You that You are a God who works even in hardship. You don't let a single event in our lives be wasted. You are constantly refining us, and this is such a blessing. I pray that as my daughters live their lives and experience inevitable difficulty, You would strengthen them in those moments and remind them You are still working. Amen.

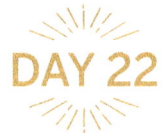

DAY 22

Patience Is Tied to Love

I therefore, a prisoner for the Lord, urge you to walk in a manner worthy of the calling to which you have been called, with all humility and gentleness, with patience, bearing with one another in love.

EPHESIANS 4:1–2

I've noticed that my daughter is not like me in a lot of ways, but there are some ways we're similar. We are not patient people. As an impatient person, I find my daughter's impatience glaringly obvious. I have this hypothesis that as humans, we notice strengths in other people that we wish we had, and we also clearly observe our own weaknesses in other people. A classic case of both positive and negative projection.

Being impatient causes a lot of internal angst. As an impatient adult, I know my impatience is not a virtue, so I try to hide it as often as possible. And as a mother, I know my daughter's impatience causes her to have big feelings that aren't always that comfortable. Patience sounds really good to me, but it is a skill that I need to work on.

These verses in Ephesians make it clear that patience is a key characteristic of how a Christian should behave. It reminds us that there is no higher calling than being a disciple of Jesus and that it is our duty to walk and talk in a way that reflects that honor. Patience is tied to love, and love is what we are called to do.

If my daughter only ever sees me giving way to my impatient nature, there's no reason she would ever try to cultivate patience in her own character. As her mother, I need to do the work of growing in patience so that she will see that people are meant to grow, not stay stuck. I also need to be willing to tell my daughter when I see impatience winning the battle in her life. She (and the people in her life) will not be served well if I don't try to help her turn from impatience to patience. As mothers, we love our daughters. Love is tied to patience, which means that together, we will work on growing that virtue.

LET'S REFLECT

- Do you identify as more of a patient person or an impatient person? What evidence backs up your assessment?
- How do you see the connection between love and patience having an impact on your mother-daughter relationship?

TAKE ACTION: Today, when you're tempted to react with impatience, take a deep breath and try something new. Model what it looks like to control your emotions and grow in character. I promise, your daughter will notice.

LET'S PRAY

Thank You for being a God who is full of mercy and grace. I ask forgiveness for the times when I'm impatient, and I ask that by the power of Your Spirit and Your transforming Word, You would help me grow in patience. I ask that You would do the same work in my daughters' hearts. I ask this in Your name. Amen.

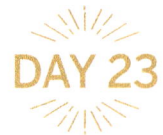

DAY 23

From Heavy to Light

*Anxiety in a man's heart weighs him down,
but a good word makes him glad.*

PROVERBS 12:25

Over the past year, we've been stuck in a 24-hour news cycle. Our minds and hearts have been weighed down by constant reports of sickness, death, racism, division, murder, hate, storms, rioting, and protests. It feels heavy.

It's an interesting thing that thoughts are invisible and technically weightless, yet they have the ability to be heavier than physical things. Humans are body, mind, and spirit. Often we think only the physical body can feel pain or weight, but it's not true. The mind and spirit can be painfully weighed down as well.

Our daughters are no exception to this, and the young, growing mind isn't able to process bad news and the subsequent anxiety in the same way that a mature mind can. As mothers, we aren't able to shield them from every bad thing that may cause them anxiety, but there are things we can do to lighten their load and make their hearts glad.

One thing we can do is be real with our daughters and tell them that the world is filled with sin, and that bad news and tragedy are part of that. We can remind our daughters that people tend to fixate on bad news and talk about it a lot, and it can turn into a cycle that compounds anxiety. Making them aware of the reality of how humans operate can help them understand why bad news often seems more prevalent than good news.

Another thing we can do is be positive, even in the midst of trials. This proverb tells us that a good word makes the heart glad. We need to point out the beauty in the world: the beauty in nature, the beauty in relationships, the kindness of our neighbors, and the love we share. We can remind our daughters of the qualities that we see God put inside them, and we can encourage our daughters in those qualities. Our words can lighten the load on their hearts and minds.

Most important of all, we can remind them that amid the uncertainty and storms of this life, we have a hope that transcends it all. God's promises are always kept, and He never changes. He will make all things new. When we speak these words of gospel truth to our daughters, we're taking away the power of anxiety and filling their hearts with beauty and promise.

LET'S REFLECT

- Have you felt the weight of all the bad news we're constantly exposed to? How does it make you feel, and how do you imagine your daughter feels?
- What is a way you deal with anxiety in your home?

TAKE ACTION: Today, when you take in the news, pick out a story to talk and pray about with your daughter. Reframe the issue through a gospel lens, and remind her of the hope that we have as believers. By doing this, you are modeling for her that we don't have to hide from reality, but we can look at reality objectively and from a gospel-centered, hope-filled perspective.

LET'S PRAY

Thank You for being our hope and our promise in the uncertainties of life. We know that the world is not perfect, and we know that the reality of it all can weigh us down. I pray that You would help my daughters and me stay focused on the truth of who You are, so that our hearts can be glad no matter the circumstances. Amen.

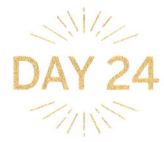

DAY 24

Temporary Home

He will wipe away every tear from their eyes, and death shall be no more, neither shall there be mourning, nor crying, nor pain anymore, for the former things have passed away.

REVELATION 21:4

One of my favorite songs is "Temporary Home" by Carrie Underwood. It's a beautiful song that reminds us that no matter where we find ourselves in life, this is only our temporary home. As good as things may be, better is on the horizon. Or as terrible as things may be, perfection is coming.

A common saying is that death is the only guarantee in this life. While that sounds morbid, it is accurate (unless Jesus returns before we die). Each one of us who breathes will one day take our last breath. Our hearts will stop beating, our blood will stop pumping, and our eyes will close for the final time. You've likely lost someone very close to you, and there's a good chance your daughter already has, too. In those moments of loss, it's hard to see any hope or joy at all. We need to consciously remind ourselves that this world, this life, is not the end.

This past year has made me look forward to heaven in a whole new way. Where I live, during COVID-19, we were forced to isolate ourselves from each other. Racial tensions were brought to new heights, and the division grew deep. Churches were forced to close, and singing with other believers was not permitted. The thought of heaven, with people of every tribe and nation gathered together worshipping God, became the most beautiful thing. I thought of my loved ones who have already passed, and I rejoiced for them, knowing that they were experiencing their true home. What we have here . . . is only temporary.

Revelation has become one of my favorite books of the Bible. The last two chapters are filled with such beautiful imagery of what is to come. Until then, though, we are in the in-between. The "already" and the "not yet." We are redeemed, and we are saved, but we are not yet living with the complete fulfillment of what is promised. One day, heaven will come down, God will be with us, and death, mourning, crying, and pain will be no more.

Create a beautiful temporary home for your daughter. Make her feel loved, teach her well, introduce her to Jesus. But most of all, remind her that this home is temporary and there is something so much better coming.

LET'S REFLECT

- How do you respond to the idea of death?
- How does it make you feel that this is your temporary home? Are you willing to let go in anticipation of what is coming?

TAKE ACTION: Listen to the song "Temporary Home" with your daughter and allow it to spark a conversation.

LET'S PRAY

Thank You, Lord, for Your Word and the promises we find inside. Thank You for being the perfect sacrifice so that we have the promise of eternal life in a home that is beyond our comprehension, yet exactly what we are meant for. I pray that my daughters would find comfort in this truth. Amen.

DAY 25
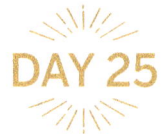
See What God Sees

But the Lord said to Samuel, "Do not look on his appearance or on the height of his stature, because I have rejected him. For the Lord sees not as man sees: man looks on the outward appearance, but the Lord looks on the heart."

1 SAMUEL 16:7

When I was growing up, we had a big Rottweiler named Tomie as our family pet. Rottweilers are big, but this one was especially big. He was muscular and athletic and weighed 140 pounds. I grew up on a farm, and this dog was our constant companion. He would race us on the ATV, and his favorite activity was chasing coyotes and, sometimes, bears. Whenever someone would drive onto our property, they would look at him in fear and not get out of their vehicle.

 The truth is, though, while Tomie appeared terrifying, he was actually a teddy bear. My siblings and I would dress him up in costumes and use him as a pillow while we watched the clouds float by. My mom and dad used to joke that if someone broke into our house or barns, Tomie wouldn't deter them at all . . . he'd likely help them carry out any expensive equipment they wanted to get their hands on. His looks were deceiving.

 In today's passage, God had to remind Samuel of that very same thing. He was there at God's request to anoint a king from among the sons of Jesse. He thought for sure it would be the eldest son, since he was tall, handsome, and strong. But God quickly corrected Samuel and told him that God sees people differently than we do. Often, we judge by what we see on the outside, but God judges based on what He sees on the inside.

Our daughters are going to be judged by what they look like on the outside, and sometimes, those judgments may hurt them. Conversely, our daughters will also likely judge others by what they see on the outside. Everyone does at some point, and usually more than once. As mothers, we must do our best to remind our daughters that their worth is not found in their size, complexion, or anything else physical. Their worth comes from being a daughter of the King, made in the image of God, and the same is true for all other people.

LET'S REFLECT

- Have you ever been judged by your appearance? Or have you judged others by their appearance?
- Why do you think it's so important for young girls to understand that the appearance of a person does not tell the whole story?

TAKE ACTION: Read today's Bible verse with your daughter. Have a discussion about what it means for God to see the heart of a person before their appearance.

LET'S PRAY

God, thank You that Your ways are higher than ours. We live in a world that likes to put a shiny veneer on the things we see, but You remind us that the heart is what matters. I pray that You would give my daughters a deep confidence that comes not from how they look but from who their God is. Amen.

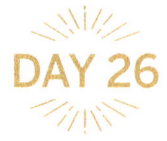

DAY 26

Worth > Worries

Look at the birds of the air: they neither sow nor reap nor gather into barns, and yet your heavenly Father feeds them. Are you not of more value than they?

MATTHEW 6:26

We live on a farm out in the country. We're surrounded by trees and mountains, and birds love it here. We'll often sit outside and watch them flying around. Birds, it seems, have a really good life. They have little societies, and it has become clear that they even have routines. We see the same birds doing the same things at the same times each morning and evening. It's pretty fascinating.

People are kind of like that. We have societies, we have routines . . . but one big difference is that the birds don't seem to be weighed down by the things we allow ourselves to be weighed down by. Though they're small, they live with a certain confidence that their every need is attended to.

God takes note of the birds; He cares for them. But we know that God has placed so much more value on us. Genesis 1:26 says, "Then God said, 'Let us make man in our image, after our likeness. And let them have dominion over the fish of the sea and over the birds of the heavens and over the livestock and over all the earth and over every creeping thing that creeps on the earth.'" There is no other piece of creation that was made in the image of God. We are highly favored, and we are wholly loved.

Our daughters need to know that they are worthy and they are cared for because they are made in the image of God. When they feel like no one sees them, remind them that God does. When they're worried about tomorrow, remember that God is holding them. When they can't see a way, remember that God always makes a way.

Every morning I hear the birds singing. I believe they're joining all of nature to worship God, who cares for them. Let's do the same.

LET'S REFLECT

- As you were reading this, were you reminded of some of your worries? How can you begin releasing those worries to the Lord?

- What are some strategies you can use to help your daughter see her worth and remember that she is cared for by our Creator?

TAKE ACTION: Today, listen to and watch the birds with your daughter. Tell her about what you read today, and tell her of her worth as a daughter of the King.

LET'S PRAY

God, I thank You that You are solidly beside us. Thank You for choosing me to be Your child and for trusting me to raise my daughters. I pray that You would open my eyes and heart to see all the ways You care for me, and I pray that You would help my daughters see the same things. I ask this in Your name. Amen.

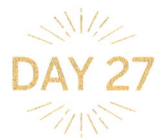

DAY 27

The Helper Is Here

Nevertheless, I tell you the truth: it is to your advantage that I go away, for if I do not go away, the Helper will not come to you. But if I go, I will send him to you.

JOHN 16:7

I often imagine what it would have been like to be a friend of Jesus when He was walking on this earth. I imagine what it would have been like to talk with Him, laugh with Him, or share a meal with Him. For me, it's hard to envision what that would have been like.

To be a friend of Jesus would have been incomparable. I can only imagine how the words from today's Bible verse must have felt falling on His friends' ears. They were probably thinking it was impossible for there to be any advantage to Jesus leaving Earth, but at the same time, they probably knew that what Jesus was saying was true . . . because every word He speaks is truth.

The Spirit that fell on the first Christians is the same Spirit that lives in each of us when we acknowledge Jesus as our Savior. In the next few verses, Jesus goes on to say what the Spirit will do. He will convict the world concerning sin, righteousness, and judgement. He says the Spirit will guide us into truth and will glorify Jesus.

What more could we ask for as parents than the Spirit guiding us into truth and convicting the world of sin? So often, we take for granted or even downplay the role of the Holy Spirit in our lives.

But Jesus wanted us to understand that the Holy Spirit would be our Helper. We aren't left to fight the battles of this world alone, and we aren't left abandoned to raise our children with just a wish and a hope. We have a Helper, and He is the Helper that Jesus was looking forward to sending.

LET'S REFLECT

- Do you feel the Holy Spirit is often downplayed or taken for granted? How so?
- Today we were reminded that the Holy Spirit is our Helper. What does that mean to you?

TAKE ACTION: Today, use your Bible concordance or the internet to search for Bible passages on the power of the Holy Spirit. Let these verses be an encouragement to you in your life and in your parenting.

LET'S PRAY

Thank You, God, for the gift that Your Son is and the gift that the Holy Spirit is. I pray that I would feel and observe the Holy Spirit at work in my life in everything I do, but particularly as I parent. I know that I cannot do it on my strength and wisdom alone but require being guided in truth by the Spirit. Thank You that You have sent the Spirit and that I'm never alone. Amen.

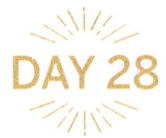

DAY 28

Forgive Like Jesus

Put on then, as God's chosen ones, holy and beloved, compassionate hearts, kindness, humility, meekness, and patience, bearing with one another and, if one has a complaint against another, forgiving each other; as the Lord has forgiven you, so you also must forgive.

COLOSSIANS 3:12–13

Forgiveness. That can be a hard thing to give. In fact, it's probably one of the very hardest things we ever give another person. There are a lot of reasons it's hard to forgive, and pride and fear are probably near the top of the list. Maybe we think forgiveness makes us look weak; it also opens us up to be hurt again by the same person.

The thing is, though, our Christian worldview is built on the backbone of forgiveness and grace. Without Christ offering us forgiveness, there would be no Christianity. There would be no hope. There would be no promise of life. We would stand forever condemned.

Jesus spoke continually of forgiveness. He healed people by saying, "Your sins are forgiven" (Matthew 9:2). He taught us to pray by forgiving others as we have been forgiven (Luke 11:4). He reminded us at the first communion that His blood was poured out for the forgiveness of sins (Matthew 26:28). And He told us to continue forgiving those who wrong us (Matthew 18:22).

As humans, we are tempted to withhold forgiveness until we see people improve their behavior. This can be true in our relationship with our daughters and others. But God doesn't operate that way. God doesn't wait for us to be perfect before He offers forgiveness. Romans 5:8 says, "But God shows his love for us in that while we were still sinners, Christ died for us." He didn't wait for the magic moment when we turned it all around. He forgave us first and then helped us turn it around.

This is what we should be modeling and doing for our daughters. There will be times when people wrong us or hurt us. We can choose how to respond. Do we choose to hold a grudge and see every imperfection? Or do we forgive and support? Christ has modeled the better way; let's put that into practice.

LET'S REFLECT

- Have you ever struggled to forgive? How did this make you feel?
- If you follow Jesus's model of forgiveness, what impact do you think this will have on your daughter?

TAKE ACTION: Take some time today to reflect on the fact that Christ died for those who He knew would continue to sin. Let that beautiful and grace-filled truth work on your heart today.

LET'S PRAY

God, You are so good and so full of grace. Thank You for forgiving me. I pray that You would help me forgive as You do, with kindness, humility, meekness, and patience. Help me bear with others rather than hold a grudge. I pray that my daughters will see You changing me and that it would change their hearts as well. Amen.

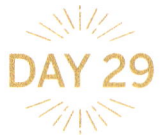

DAY 29

A Gospel-Centered Life

For what does it profit a man to gain the whole world and forfeit his soul?

MARK 8:36

Two of my kids recently went to day camp. It was five days, and we'd pick them up at the end of each day. Our six-year-old daughter wasn't old enough to go yet, so she stayed home with my husband and me. She was SO disappointed that she couldn't go. The first day was a lot of moping, but then after that, she just really started to get competitive. She wanted to make sure she had better days at home than the boys were having at camp.

Each day when we picked the boys up, she would immediately tell them all the good things she did that day and then do her best to insist that everything *she* did was better than everything *they* did. They got tired of engaging in that conversation and started to ignore her. At times, they became frustrated with her. Usually, by the time we got home, the boys tried to distance themselves from her. In her mind, she had won the battle over who had the "best day," but she'd lost her playmates. You might say that she gained the "world" but lost much more.

This is often true for adults as well. We do our best to keep up with the Joneses and end up digging ourselves into a pit of debt. Or we worry so much about how we will be perceived that we turn the opinions of others into an idol. Maybe we convince ourselves that a little more money will be the answer to our problems, but instead, it leads to our downfall. Maybe we hide our faith to save face and find ourselves opposing God.

It's uncomfortable to follow Jesus. He tells us in verse 34 of the same chapter to deny ourselves, pick up our cross, and follow Him. He never promised us that it would be easy, but He did promise that it would be worth it. We want our daughters to see what it means to live a life that is focused on the gospel above all else. Our goal as parents should be for our daughters to live that same gospel-centered life. Anything besides that is a forfeit of our very souls.

LET'S REFLECT

- What stuck out most to you from today's reading?
- How can you shift your daughter's focus from the things of this world to the things of God?

TAKE ACTION: Today, make a commitment to a routine that will put God before things of the world. Perhaps that will be committing to a routine of family devotions, service in your community, or praying together at a certain time each day—whatever would be most beneficial for your family.

LET'S PRAY

Lord, forgive me when I choose things of the world over You. I pray that You would stoke a desire within me to follow Your way above all others and to take my daughters along on that journey. I pray that You would work in our hearts and that the fruit of that would be seen in our lives. Amen.

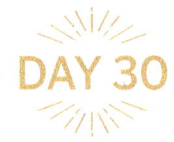

DAY 30

The Gift of Wisdom

The one who gets wisdom loves life; the one who cherishes understanding will soon prosper.

PROVERBS 19:8 NIV

In 1 Kings 3, God comes to Solomon in a dream and asks what he wants. God is willing to give him whatever he asks for. *Whoa* am I right? Part of me thinks I would love to be asked that question, and part of me would be terrified to have God ask me that question. Lucky for me, if that ever does happen, I can follow Solomon's example. Solomon, though he is young, makes an excellent request. A request that, according to 1 Kings 3:10, "pleased the Lord." Solomon asked for wisdom.

Could you imagine being young and set in charge of not just a large nation but God's chosen people? Many young people would have asked for wealth or long life, but David's son Solomon asked for wisdom. Solomon knew that he wasn't equipped to handle a kingdom on his own. He knew that he needed help from the Lord, so he put aside thoughts of his own comfort and asked for wisdom straight from God.

God was so pleased with Solomon's request that He decided to also give him riches, honor, and a long life. Today's Bible verse from Proverbs mirrors this story. It says that the one who cherishes understanding will soon prosper. This doesn't mean that we'll become millionaires or have our every want taken care of. What it does mean is that we will discover what *good* truly is. We will discover what *prosperity* truly is. Not from a worldly mindset but from a *heavenly* one.

As we raise our daughters, we need to ask for wisdom. God may not come to us in a dream like He did with Solomon, but He still wants us to ask for wisdom, and we need to heed that call.

LET'S REFLECT

- If God asked you what you wanted, what would you ask for, and why?
- As you have grown in wisdom, what is one thing God has revealed to you?

TAKE ACTION: Today, ask your daughter what she would like to ask God for. Have fun with this question. Chances are (if she's anything like my young daughter), she'll want to ask for a stuffed bunny or a pony. Laugh with her, and imagine together how wonderful her request would be if it came true. Then shift the conversation to tell her about Solomon's request. Plant the seed for her to grow in wisdom.

LET'S PRAY

God, thank You for who You are. Your thoughts are above mine, and You so graciously offer to provide me with wisdom if I ask. I'm asking You today for wisdom. As I raise my daughters, I pray that You would equip me with wisdom to raise them in Your ways, to know right from wrong and truth from lies. Thank You for loving us. Amen.

DAY 31

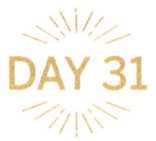

Give It Your All

But King David said to Ornan, "No, but I will buy them for the full price. I will not take for the Lord what is yours, nor offer burnt offerings that cost me nothing."

1 CHRONICLES 21:24

My daughter really loves her great-grandma. A LOT. Each day, she asks if she can go see her. I love that she wants to spend time with her (and let's be real, she also wants the candy great-grandma has on hand), but I also want to make sure we respect great-grandma's privacy.

My daughter has caught on to my hesitancy in letting her have unfettered access to her great-grandma. She's clever, though, and discovered that if she makes a gift for great-grandma, I'm more likely to let her go over there.

A few days ago, my daughter once again asked whether she could go see great-grandma, and she promised to color a picture as a gift to her. I agreed and helped her get her coloring page and supplies ready. A short few minutes later, she declared that she was done and ready to go see great-grandma. Suspicious, I asked to see the picture she had colored.

My daughter, who is usually quite particular in her coloring, had only done some quick scribbles across the page. She knew she had been caught and quickly volunteered to color a new picture. I explained to her that I knew she was in a hurry to see great-grandma, but that didn't mean she should compromise the quality of the gift she was bringing.

That is exactly what King David was getting at in today's passage. He had sinned and wanted to make an altar for an offering to the Lord. He went to a specific field, and the man offered to give it to him. David refused and instead insisted that he should pay full price. He knew that an offering to the Lord that cost him nothing would not be much of an offering at all.

Now, my daughter wasn't offering her picture to the Lord, but it provided the perfect training ground to tell my daughter this story and to weave it into the greater context of our whole lives. My life and hers are meant to be lived for the Lord. Life isn't meant to always be convenient and easy . . . there are going to be times when we have to be ready to make sacrifices that cost us something.

On the days you're feeling overwhelmed by the weight of parenting, or when your daughter is worn down by some of the challenges of life (or the thought of carefully coloring a whole picture), remind yourself and her that your lives are a living sacrifice. While that's not always comfortable, it is a blessing.

LET'S REFLECT

- What was your initial response to hearing David say that he didn't want to offer a sacrifice that cost him nothing?
- When you reflect on your own life, what sacrifices have you already made for your family and for faith?

TAKE ACTION: Today, when you're doing the chore you detest most (for me it's cleaning the shower), thank God that you get the opportunity to do it. Remember that, by serving and sacrificing for your family, you're serving and sacrificing for the Lord as well.

LET'S PRAY

God, You have given me so much. Sometimes, I get so comfortable with all the good gifts You've given me that I become stubborn and unwilling to make sacrifices. Help me remember that it's a privilege to sacrifice for my family, and especially for you. Amen.

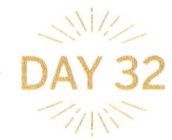

DAY 32

You Are His

But now thus says the Lord, he who created you, O Jacob, he who formed you, O Israel: "Fear not, for I have redeemed you; I have called you by name, you are mine. When you pass through the waters, I will be with you; and through the rivers, they shall not overwhelm you; when you walk through fire you shall not be burned, and the flame shall not consume you. For I am the Lord your God, the Holy One of Israel, your Savior."

ISAIAH 43:1–3

For each of our kids, we picked a life verse when they were born. This is the verse that we picked for our second child. When my first child was born, I still had a pretty rosy outlook on how his life would be. But by the time my second child was born, I was a couple of years older and had what felt like a lifetime more of personal experience. That is why we picked this verse.

What I've learned is that life is not easy. There are storms. The waters rage, and the fires burn hot. As much as I'd like to believe my children will be exempt from those hard things, I know they won't. They are human, and they live in a fallen world. They're not exempt from bad things.

While these verses may make some people fearful of the challenges that they will inevitably face in life, I feel strong when I read them. But not because I'm strong . . . because God is strong. The imagery of these verses paints a picture of a faithful God. A God who chose you before the foundation of the world. If you are a believer, God saw you as redeemed before you called on Him . . . because He knew you would.

In these verses, we see God standing beside us when the waters threaten to overwhelm us. We see Him pulling us from the fire when the flames are trying to consume us. I feel strong when I read these verses, because He is beside me.

I want all my kids to feel this same strength. That is why we chose this verse as a life verse. It doesn't promise a false reality of empty happiness, but it does promise our Redeemer beside us every step of the way. That's the true reality that I want my kids to know.

LET'S REFLECT

- How does it make you feel when you imagine your child going through challenges in life?
- What difference do you think it would make if, rather than shielding your child from the hardships of life, you introduced them to their Redeemer?

TAKE ACTION: If you haven't picked a life verse for your daughter, do that today! Then read it with her and explain why you picked it. Give her the opportunity to ask questions about it.

LET'S PRAY

God, I thank You that in this turbulent world, You are my rock and my redeemer. Thank You for Your promise to walk beside us through anything we face in life. I pray that my daughters will know You deeply and that they will feel strong because of who You are. Amen.

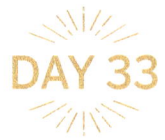

DAY 33

Doubts Are Welcome

Immediately the father of the child cried out and said, "I believe; help my unbelief!"

MARK 9:24

Does "doubt" sound like a dirty word to you? Let me assure you that it definitely isn't. There's a huge percentage of young adults leaving the church right now. Many of them are doing so because they have doubts. Wait a minute . . . I guess that doesn't sound very reassuring. Stick with me, though; I promise that the reassurance is coming.

While that's a troubling statistic, we shouldn't run from it. Knowledge is power, and this knowledge is indicating that as a church, we don't know how to properly handle doubt. As a parent, though, you're uniquely positioned to help the youth of today learn how to deal with doubt.

Today's Bible verse features a father who is desperate for Jesus's help. The man's child was besieged by an unclean spirit and was constantly suffering because of it. This father said something I could imagine so many of us saying. He said, "But if you can do anything, have compassion on us and help him." A simple, anguished request from a father hurting deeply from watching his child suffer.

Jesus's response, though, isn't to immediately heal the child. He first addresses something with the father. The father had said, "If you can." Jesus wanted to know whether he really believed. The father was in anguish as he replied, "I believe; help my unbelief!" This father didn't put on any pretenses. He didn't act as if he had his faith all figured out. He didn't button up his emotions and keep them in a neat and tidy box. He poured out the truth to Jesus.

He believed . . . but he needed help with the part of him that still didn't believe. Do you know what that's called? Doubt.

The beautiful thing is that Jesus didn't condemn the man for his doubts. He also didn't question him relentlessly about why he had doubts. Jesus simply allowed the man to be honest, and then He healed his son.

Just like you have doubts sometimes, so will your daughter. Learn to love the conversations where you explore doubt together. Let her know that it's okay to have doubts, that she's not the only person to doubt, and that you're a safe person to talk to about those doubts. As you talk about doubt together, use it as an opportunity to learn together. Dig into some apologetics (the defense of the Christian faith), and let your faith grow right alongside your daughter's. Teach her that doubt is not a dirty word and that you're always a safe person to talk with.

LET'S REFLECT

- Do you feel safe to express or admit doubt? Why or why not?
- How does it make you feel to consider having conversations with your daughter about faith and doubt?

TAKE ACTION: Reflect on doubts you have or have had about your faith and what you have learned from those doubts. If your daughter is old enough to have that conversation, explain to her what you learned.

LET'S PRAY

I thank You that You are a patient God and that You don't scoff or turn Your back when I face doubt. I see so many young people struggling with their doubt and not knowing what to do about it. I pray that You would make me a safe place for my daughters to discuss doubt. May we grow closer to You and to each other as we learn more about You. Amen.

DAY 34

Know His Ways

Teach me your way, O Lord, that I may walk in your truth; unite my heart to fear your name.

PSALM 86:11

As our daughters grow, they're going to find themselves going from the comfort and safety of our homes to being independent. While they were living with us, we could protect, guide, direct, and catch them when they stumbled. But one day soon, they're going to fledge from the nest. Before they take flight, they'll probably look out at the big wide world and wonder whether they're really ready.

As moms, we'll be standing behind them as they consider taking flight. We'll have done everything we can to raise them right, and despite our own worries, we'll be attempting to send them off with confidence. How can we know that they're truly ready? How can we know that the foundation we provided was firm and lasting?

Each day, I pray the same words. I ask God that my kids would know Him, love Him, and serve Him their whole lives. This is my most frequent prayer. I truly believe that if our kids know God, they will ultimately be okay, no matter what life throws at them. I believe that truly knowing God is the only way to be equipped for the future.

Today's Bible verse addresses that. It's a prayer: a really important prayer. It says, "Teach me your way, O Lord." We should be praying that for ourselves but also for our daughters. Ask God to teach your daughter His ways. Believe that when He does, she will always walk in His truth. His truth is the only place we want our daughters walking.

The verse goes on to say, "Unite my heart to fear your name." By saying "unite" in this psalm, King David is saying that we don't want just a piece of our hearts to be carefully following after the Lord. We require our whole heart to follow after the Lord.

One day, our daughters will fly from the nest. This is a good thing; it's what we've been preparing them for. Education is important. Friendships are important. But above all, help build your daughter a truly firm foundation. Help her know the Lord, and teach her to continue praying that the Lord would show her more about who He is and reveal the way that she can walk in His truth.

LET'S REFLECT

- When you consider your daughter growing up and leaving home, what concerns you the most, and why?
- Have you made praying for your daughter a consistent habit? What could you do to grow in this area?

TAKE ACTION: Begin a practice of praying daily that your daughter would know the Lord, love Him, and serve Him. Start today, and commit to continuing this practice.

LET'S PRAY

God, I thank You that You care for us, and I thank You that You are a lamp to our feet. I pray that as my daughters grow, You would teach them Your ways. Reveal Your truth, and keep their path well lit as they walk in Your truth. May You take their whole hearts and mold them to be constantly in pursuit of You. Amen.

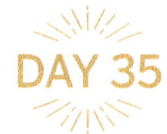

DAY 35

What Love Is and Isn't

Love is patient and kind; love does not envy or boast; it is not arrogant or rude. It does not insist on its own way; it is not irritable or resentful; it does not rejoice at wrongdoing, but rejoices with the truth. Love bears all things, believes all things, hopes all things, endures all things.

1 CORINTHIANS 13:4–7

Oooh boy. This passage in 1 Corinthians has always been so compelling to me. You see, I'm the type of person who's efficient, fairly particular, and rather impatient. Don't I sound so fun? This passage does such a thorough job of describing what love is and what love isn't, and each time I read it, I'm reminded that there are a few things I need to work on when it comes to love.

In fact, I was so compelled by this passage that I got a tattoo of a portion of it on my forearm, along with a large cross. It's a daily reminder that I don't have love all figured out. And trust me, I need that daily reminder.

For example, my daughter loves to play this imaginary game with me called Lost and Found Kitty. I do not like imaginary games . . . I'm pretty sure I didn't even like them as a child. Every time she asks me to play it with her, I want to say no. But then I remember that love is patient and kind (unlike me), and I say yes. Not every time, but often enough. I say yes, and she transforms into a lost kitten who was abandoned. I find her and welcome her into my home. It's always the same, but it always makes her feel loved.

I also need to be reminded about the qualities of love when I'm cleaning up discarded laundry for the millionth time, or flushing the toilet for the eighteenth time that day since it seems no one else can remember. I need to remember what love is.

On top of that, though, it's our responsibility as mothers to help our kids learn how to love. So while I need to be patient about the scattered laundry, the messy house, and the unflushed toilets, I need to help my kids learn that making an effort to do those things themselves is a way that they can show love. Love is something that we have to teach while we're still learning.

A mother who is intent on growing in love is a mother who will raise daughters intent on growing in love. It may not be easy, but it is so worth it.

LET'S REFLECT

- Do you struggle with any of these characteristics of love? If so, which ones do you need to work on?
- As you see your daughter interact with others (maybe siblings, friends, or other family members), do you notice her exhibiting the qualities of love? Have you encouraged that behavior?

TAKE ACTION: Write out today's scripture passage and hang it in a prominent location in your home. Begin memorizing it and encouraging your daughter to do the same.

LET'S PRAY

God, I thank You that You are a God of perfect love. Thank You for Your patience as we stumble along doing our best to learn how to love and to teach our children to love. I pray that You would change our hearts to be more like Yours, full of gracious, merciful love. Amen.

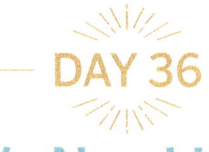

DAY 36

We Need Him

The God who made the world and everything in it, being Lord of heaven and earth, does not live in temples made by man, nor is he served by human hands, as though he needed anything, since he himself gives to all mankind life and breath and everything.

ACTS 17:24–25

Why do we serve God? Why do we worship Him? How often do you take the time to stop and consider who this God is whom you have given your life to? Has it become a habit to serve Him, or is it something you do because you realize in the core of your being who He is and what He is worthy of?

As we live our lives, raise our kids, and serve in our churches and communities, it can all begin to feel really routine. Not only that, but we begin to worry that if we weren't doing the things we're doing, everything would crumble. I believe it's a common problem in our modern times that in the midst of all we've been given, we forget that God doesn't need us. We need Him.

That's why I love today's Bible verses. In the midst of our busy, crammed lives, they serve as a reminder that God is bigger than the things we toil away at. God created the whole world and everything in it. We can't put Him in a little box, or in a building, and all the busy work in the world that we do is not needed by Him. I mean, really—He created the universe, and we think He needs us?

He doesn't. So then why does He bother with us? Love. He bothers with us because He loves us. We don't serve Him because we have to; we serve Him because we want to. A few verses later, in verse 28, Paul says, "In him we live and move and have our being."

Our very breath comes from Him. Every move we make is allowed by Him, and every action we take. As we raise our daughters, we need to keep this truth in perspective. God doesn't need us, but He chooses us, loves us, and empowers us. It is a gift to serve Him in whatever way He has called us to, especially in motherhood.

LET'S REFLECT

- What stood out most to you from today's reading?
- Do you often or rarely reflect on the fact that every breath we have is a gift from the Creator of the universe?

TAKE ACTION: Today, listen to some worship songs that talk about the greatness of God. Reflect on the lyrics. Examples of songs include "How Great Thou Art," "How Great Is Our God," "Indescribable," and "The Lion and the Lamb." There are so many more!

LET'S PRAY

God, You are so great. I pray that You would affect my heart with Your majesty. Remind me that I serve the Creator of the oceans, the mountains, the stars, the planets, myself, and my daughters. I pray that as I'm struck by Your glory, I would pour my heart and soul into serving You—not because You need me, but because You love me. Amen.

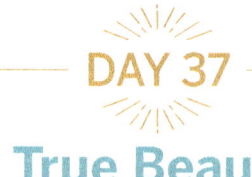

DAY 37

True Beauty

Charm is deceitful, and beauty is vain, but a woman who fears the Lord is to be praised.

PROVERBS 31:30

My daughter has beautiful, thick, blonde, shiny hair. By the time she was five, her hair had grown past her waist. She looked a little bit like Rapunzel from the movie *Tangled*.

One night, just a couple of weeks after her fifth birthday, my husband and I put the kids to bed and were watching a show. We thought the kids had gone to sleep, because the house was quiet. We were wrong, though. So very wrong.

All of a sudden, the kids came bounding into the living room with looks of pride on their sweet faces. My husband and I were hit with shock and confusion as we looked at our daughter. She stood before us in her too-short Ariel pajamas missing about 18 inches of hair. With the help of her brothers, she had chopped off her iconic hair. I may sound dramatic when I call her hair iconic . . . but it was. It was what everyone talked about when they met her or saw her.

Her hair got fixed up the next morning by a hairstylist, and she went from long Rapunzel locks to a Tinkerbell pixie cut. People would still comment on her beauty . . . that was unchanged. However, the epic haircut of 2020 caused a shift inside of my husband and me. We had to come to terms with the fact that we had a strong emotional attachment to her long hair; it seemed to be intrinsically tied to her personality. But it wasn't. Her personality was just as fiery and passionate post-haircut as it was pre-haircut. It was completely untouched by the scissors that cut her hair.

While my daughter didn't learn much of a lesson from cutting her hair (she cut it again a couple of weeks later), I did. It was a great reminder that her beauty doesn't come from her appearance. Yes, she is physically beautiful, but the best part of her comes from inside. Longer hair wouldn't make her more beautiful, but a heart that sought after God would always be the most beautiful thing about her.

The same is true for you and your daughter as well. True beauty is not based on outward appearances (1 Peter 3:3) but on the Spirit inside.

LET'S REFLECT

- The world prizes physical beauty. Do you ever get physical beauty mixed up with true beauty?
- Do you have concerns about your daughter being duped into thinking her appearance matters more than what's on the inside?

TAKE ACTION: Make a point of complimenting your daughter on her character today. That could be her patience, kindness, gentleness, and so on. Make a habit of encouraging her on the beauty that comes from within.

LET'S PRAY

God, I thank You that You see the heart so much more clearly than I do. I pray that You would open my eyes to see the beauty in people the way You do, and that You would do likewise for my daughters. I pray that they would see themselves as beautiful because You are their Father. Amen.

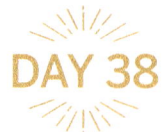

DAY 38

The Real Battleground

For though we walk in the flesh, we are not waging war according to the flesh. For the weapons of our warfare are not of the flesh but have divine power to destroy strongholds. We destroy arguments and every lofty opinion raised against the knowledge of God, and take every thought captive to obey Christ.

2 CORINTHIANS 10:3–5

I don't know about you, but as a mom raising kids, I don't like to think of the fact that we're in a war. I want to believe that everything is peaceful and quiet. But that's not the reality. This isn't the kind of war where soldiers are shipped off for training and they experience grueling mental and physical challenges to prepare them for the realities of war. This isn't the kind of battle where we arm ourselves with weaponry and plot out our strategies. But preparation is still important.

  The battleground that we're facing as Christian moms is a battle for the hearts and minds of all people . . . especially our children. Our kids aren't bystanders, either. They're engaged in the same battle, and it's our job to teach them what the battle is about and how to fight.

  The battle is about truth, God, and the gospel. It can be tricky, though, because this battle usually gets muddied by cultural issues. The cultural issues become the face of the battle, and it can appear as if that's what the battle is about. But we have to know that those things are only on the surface. The true battle is at the core of these issues, and that is the battle over truth, God, and the gospel.

Now that we know what the battle is about, we have to know how to fight it and how to teach our kids to fight it. We fight by knowing the truth, and we know the truth by reading the scripture and praying. The weapons of prayer and scripture are so much better than weapons of the flesh, because they are powered by God, and they empower us. When we prepare and fight the battle in this way, we won't get so easily confused by the cultural issues that form the face of the battle.

Amid this battle, our thoughts and our daughters' thoughts will face moments of challenge. We will wonder whether what we're doing is right. In those moments, we need to take our thoughts captive and look to Christ. Go back to prayer, go back to scripture . . . and walk in truth.

LET'S REFLECT

- Which cultural issue is the face of the battle you're currently fighting?
- In moments of confusion, do you struggle to take your thoughts captive?

TAKE ACTION: Identify the battles that are going on around you. Rather than trying to ignore or gloss over them, engage with them through prayer and reading the scripture. Take your thoughts and worries captive, bring them to Christ, and form an opinion on the issue based on the truth of what the Lord says.

LET'S PRAY

God, I thank You that You are watching over us and haven't left us to fight the battles of this world on our own. Thank You for hearing my prayers and for providing a guide via Your Word. I pray that in this confusing cultural moment, You would help me fight for the hearts and minds of my daughters, and I pray that You would show me Your truth more clearly each day. Amen.

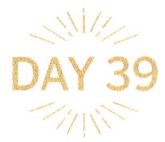

DAY 39

The Joy in Trials

Count it all joy, my brothers, when you meet trials of various kinds, for you know that the testing of your faith produces steadfastness.

JAMES 1:2–3

Today's Bible verses say that joy and trials are not mutually exclusive; they can be linked. I learned that in early 2020. My son was sick, and I will forever remember it as one of the scariest times of my life. We were in the middle of a days-long blizzard. Leading up to his diagnosis and hospitalization, my husband had to bring him back and forth to the hospital a couple of times. Each time they had to do this it was dark, windy, and snowy. I would watch my husband drive out of the driveway, pedal to the metal trying to push through snowdrifts, and then watch the lights disappear into the swirling snow.

Despite our worries and frequent trips to the hospital, they kept sending my son home. On the third trip to the hospital, they got him in quickly and admitted him with pneumonia. I was home with the other two kids. It was so difficult not to be with my sick son, and I was plagued with worry and doubt. That night, I got multiple people praying and then went to bed with worship music on. Somehow, in the midst of my worries and doubts, my heart was thankful and joyful. I was able to do what I thought would be impossible: I slept.

In the morning, I got a call from my husband, who was following the ambulance with my son in it as they transferred him to a bigger hospital with better pediatric care, because they were having trouble managing his oxygen levels and symptoms. Within a couple of hours, my pastor had picked me up, and we were on the road to see my son. Four days later, we were back home, and he has been healthy ever since.

As I write this, tears still come to my eyes. I never want to repeat that, or God forbid, go through worse, but I know that if I do, it won't be wasted pain. Through that time, God held me close. My faith was tested, and He carried me. He brought me peace, and when it seemed impossible, He filled me with joy.

God offers the same to you. You will face trials, and so will your daughter. Your faith will be tested, but you can know that God is working through it all. And that should be counted as joy.

LET'S REFLECT

- What resonated most with you from today's reading?
- Have you been able to find joy and growth through challenges? Why or why not?

TAKE ACTION: Reflect on one of the big challenges you've faced in life. Examine how your faith was tested and how you grew through it. Let this exercise encourage you through any future challenge you may face.

LET'S PRAY

Thank You, God, for walking with me through everything that this life brings. Thank You for the good days and the bad days, and the fact You use all my days to refine me and bring me closer to You. I pray that You would help my daughters find the same joy in trials, knowing You are beside them all the way. Amen.

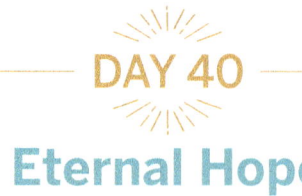

DAY 40
Eternal Hope

For we know that if the tent that is our earthly home is destroyed, we have a building from God, a house not made with hands, eternal in the heavens.

2 CORINTHIANS 5:1

Lately, I've become quite interested in the topic of bio-digital convergence. If you haven't heard of it, it's essentially exactly what it sounds like. It's the merging of a living being with artificial intelligence. I could ask five people their opinion on this topic, and each person would likely have a different response. But for me . . . it makes me think of where our hope is found.

    The big drivers for proponents of this technology seem to be two things: For the creators of the technology, the driver is profits (obviously). For the public, it's fear. The 2020 pandemic has been like kindling in a fire for the growth of this technology, because people have become so fearful of death. This bio-digital technology promises a generally hands-off society, which means less pathogen spread and more monitoring of your personal health and comfort by AI.

    While this technology is stoking the hopes of many people for a healthier, safer, longer life, it's inducing sadness in me. Sadness, because people have placed their hope in technology. People have become so bent on preserving their lives that they're willing to sacrifice their social lives, their privacy, and face-to-face human interaction. To me, this isn't *hope-filled* but *hopeless*.

    From a Christian perspective, hope is felt because we know that the earth and our bodies are not perfect, but that we're promised an eternal home in the heavens. Not a shoddy version of eternal life manufactured in a lab, but eternal life crafted and promised by the Creator of the universe. As you raise up your daughter, raise her to be bold in her hope. Raise her not to fear but to look forward with confidence, because the best is yet to come.

LET'S REFLECT

- Have you heard of bio-digital convergence before? Does it fill you with more hope than what is promised by our Savior?
- From a Christian perspective, what gives you confidence for your daughter's future?

TAKE ACTION: Read Psalm 130 today as a supplement to today's Bible verse. Be encouraged in hope.

LET'S PRAY

God, I thank You that the eternity You promise us is not limited, isolated, or driven by fear. I thank You that You promise abundance and joy and restoration. I pray that You will help me raise my daughters to be filled with boldness and hope and that they will live in anticipation of the promises You have made. Amen.

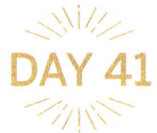

DAY 41

Creation's Sermon

The heavens declare the glory of God, and the sky above proclaims his handiwork. Day to day pours out speech, and night to night reveals knowledge. There is no speech, nor are there words, whose voice is not heard. Their voice goes out through all the earth, and their words to the end of the world. In them he has set a tent for the sun, which comes out like a bridegroom leaving his chamber, and, like a strong man, runs its course with joy. Its rising is from the end of the heavens, and its circuit to the end of them, and there is nothing hidden from its heat.

PSALM 19:1–6

Over the next two days, we're going to be looking at Psalm 19 together. This is one of my favorite psalms, and every time I see a sunset decorating the sky, this passage comes to mind. God reveals Himself through two methods. Method 1 is general revelation, which is what we observe through nature and the created world. Method 2 is through special revelation, which is the Word of God. Today, with these first six verses of Psalm 19, we're focusing on general revelation.

Over time, humanity has evolved from living outdoors in primitive shelters. Our homes have become so comfortable that we rarely feel the need to go out in nature.

King David wrote Psalm 19, and as I read his words, I'm struck by the realization that this was a man who not only spent time outside but was in awe when he observed the beauty and complexity of creation. He didn't see nature as static or silent but as dynamic and vocal. Through his poetic words, he puts forth the idea that creation is revealing God's glory . . . even preaching.

God created us, mind, body, and spirit. We're not simply a brain, or just a brain and a soul. We are physical with bodies. We are part of creation, and we are meant to enjoy creation. We aren't meant to simply run from car to house, store, or school. We are meant to take the time to see what God has revealed about Himself through nature.

Our daughters are going to be tempted (as we are) to take nature for granted. They (like us) are going to spend many hours indoors. As moms, we need to take our duty seriously to help our daughters see the wonders of God, and to encourage them to go outside and breathe in the glory of what God has surrounded us with. By doing this, we will be contributing to their health ... the health of their mind, body, and spirit.

LET'S REFLECT

- Do you take the time to get out into God's creation? Why or why not?
- How do you feel when you allow yourself the time and space to simply "be" outdoors?

TAKE ACTION: Today, make time to get outside with your daughter. When you do, avoid bringing your phone or any other digital distractions if you can. Just breathe deeply and observe the landscape, listen to the birds, soak in some sun, and feel the breeze. Your body, mind, and soul will thank you for it.

LET'S PRAY

God, You are so great. I look around at Your creation in awesome wonder. I'm humbled by the complexity and beauty of Your creation, and I'm honored to not only be part of it but to bear Your image within it. I pray that my daughters would draw peace, comfort, and confidence from Your creation as well, and that through it, You would draw them closer to You. Amen.

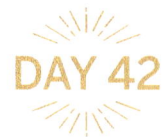

DAY 42

The Word of Life

The law of the Lord is perfect, reviving the soul; the testimony of the Lord is sure, making wise the simple; the precepts of the Lord are right, rejoicing the heart; the commandment of the Lord is pure, enlightening the eyes; the fear of the Lord is clean, enduring forever; the rules of the Lord are true, and righteous altogether. More to be desired are they than gold, even much fine gold; sweeter also than honey and drippings of the honeycomb. Moreover, by them is your servant warned; in keeping them there is great reward.

PSALM 19:7–11

Yesterday we talked about how God reveals Himself to us through nature. Today, we're digging into how He reveals Himself through His Word. The general revelation of creation is such a blessing; it's a blessing aesthetically, spiritually, and even physically. While it's such an important part of God's revelation to us, it doesn't specifically reveal Jesus Christ and the redemption He has offered us.

But the special revelation of the Bible *does* reveal Jesus Christ to us. As we're raising our daughters to know the Lord, we have to equip them and train them with the biggest tool God gave us: His Word.

Psalm 19 tells us what God's Word does for us. We live in a world where our souls grow weary, but God's Word revives our souls. His Word causes our hearts to rejoice, and it opens our eyes. His Word is eternal, unchanging, perfect, and the only source of truth. These are beautiful things that we want for our daughters.

The truth is, though, the Bible is often pushed aside in favor of Instagram stories, TikTok videos, and the algorithms of Netflix and YouTube, which sometimes seem to know us better than we know ourselves. We, and our daughters, have become accustomed to high-definition images and quick sound bites, and it can feel unnatural to sit quietly with the Bible and its simple white pages filled with little black words.

Psalm 19 says that the words, rules, and precepts of the Lord are to be desired above all. It says that they're sweeter than honey and finer than gold. But it seems so many of us have lost sight of this vital truth. So what do we do? How can we help our daughters see the value of the Word of God?

First, we model what it looks like to love the Word. We go to it daily for wisdom and refreshment. We invite our daughters to join us in our study and enjoyment of the Word . . . and we pray. We pray that God would stir in our daughters' hearts a desire to know Him more, and we believe that God is listening and responding.

LET'S REFLECT

- What impacted you most from today's reading?
- Do you prize God's Word as highly as King David did? If not, what has gotten in the way?

TAKE ACTION: Begin committing these few verses to memory. When other things compete to take the place of God's Word in your life or the life of your family, use this passage to remind you of the solid foundation the Word gives to your life.

LET'S PRAY

Thank You, Lord, for Your Word. It is a spring of pure water that brings life to my weary soul. I pray that You would help me prize it higher than any of the things of earth and that my daughters would prize it in that same way. Amen.

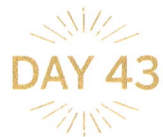

DAY 43

The Suffering Servant

Do nothing from selfish ambition or conceit, but in humility count others more significant than yourselves. Let each of you look not only to his own interests, but also to the interests of others.

PHILIPPIANS 2:3–4

It has been quite the morning in the Dickey house. We're in the middle of what very much seems to be a drought. Which is an odd thing when you live in a temperate coniferous rain forest. Usually, we have the mildest temperatures in all of Canada, and the most fertile ground. But this summer has been so hot, and we haven't had any rain. My apple trees are dying in the front yard, my garden looks a bit limp and sickly, and our usually soft, green grass is now brown and prickly.

As irritable as the vegetation is feeling, humans are feeling it, too. While my kids aren't perfect, they usually don't fight much. But lately, and I'm blaming this on the heat, they're really getting on each other's nerves. One wants to watch a TV show. The other wants to play with one sibling but not the other. The third is pretending to feel left out, but my mom-senses tell me he doesn't actually care about being excluded, he just wants to make an issue out of things. Overall, it's a fun time as each of my children pushes for their own agenda and refuses to even entertain the idea of having respectful dialogue with their siblings.

Case in point, humans really are a selfish species. Left to our own devices, it seems we will fight for our own fulfillment above all else. But the gospel tells a different story. Jesus left his throne in heaven to come to the dirt of the earth. He wasn't born to a king but to a carpenter and a rumor-wrought virgin. He didn't rise to power like many would expect of a king, but instead He bent low to serve. He didn't protect His life at all costs, but instead laid down His life to save the souls of all who would listen.

The gospel isn't about bettering our own lives. The gospel teaches us that though we are unworthy, we are counted worthy because of Jesus. The gospel is filled with grace, yet it convicts us to put others ahead of ourselves. This is not an easy lesson, but it is a lesson we have to help our daughters learn.

Our job is to show them Jesus, the suffering servant. He is our model of a life well-lived.

LET'S REFLECT

- Compare and contrast the posture of Jesus to the basics of human nature. What differences do you see?
- What is one way you can help your daughter elevate others?

TAKE ACTION: Read this passage with your daughter today, and talk about the example that Jesus has set for us. Discuss how we don't model ourselves after His behavior because we have to but because we are thankful for what He has done for us.

LET'S PRAY

God, I thank You for sending Your Son. Christ died for us. He showed humility in His life, death, and resurrection. I pray that You would convict my heart to take on those same characteristics. Help me show my daughters that by serving others, we're serving Jesus. Amen.

DAY 44
Stay Awake

*So then let us not sleep, as others do, but
let us keep awake and be sober.*

1 THESSALONIANS 5:6

Okay, let's get one thing straight before we start. I'm not proposing you literally stay awake and never sleep. I'm a big fan of sleep. So much so that even though my husband doesn't snore, I wear earplugs at night. He breathes, and that's enough to annoy me when I'm tired. So, I think sleep is good. Very, very good.

Alright, now that we've gotten that disclaimer out of the way, we can proceed!

There's nothing that motivates me as a mother more than thinking of my child's eternity. I know . . . that just went from earplugs to intense real quick. Sorry about that. But I'm thankful for passages like this one from 1 Thessalonians because they keep me from getting complacent and distracted.

We love to be distracted. There are entire industries built around the fact that humans like to choose distraction over the hard things in life. Algorithms have been perfected to keep us lulled into a comfortable and entertaining state of distraction. But here's the thing: Distraction kills. Maybe not right away. It's insidious and sneaky, and it preys on our weaknesses. For a mother who is raising eternal souls, distraction is a tool of the enemy.

When Paul is writing in this letter to the Thessalonians to stay awake, he's calling on them to not fall asleep at the spiritual wheel. He's reminding them that they have been trusted with ONE life, and he's reminding us that through Christ we've been given a gift that is not to be wasted. He's also reminding us that through Christ we have been equipped to stay spiritually awake.

This world is not forever. Tomorrow is not guaranteed. But God has a promise for those who are in Christ. He has a promise for those who stay awake and sober-minded. That promise is what I want for my daughter and all my children. Because of that, I will lift my life up as an offering. I will stay awake. And I encourage you to do the same.

LET'S REFLECT

- How do you feel when you are reminded of eternity?
- What do you imagine it looks like to stay "awake"?

TAKE ACTION: Read through all of 1 Thessalonians 5:1–11 and study the passage.

LET'S PRAY

Thank You, Lord, for Your patience. Thank You for Your Word and Your faithful reminders that this life is temporary and not to be wasted. Thank You for Your promise of eternity with Jesus. I pray that You would grab hold of my daughters' hearts. Hold them close to You, now and for all eternity. Amen.

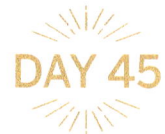

DAY 45

There's Always a Way Out

No temptation has overtaken you that is not common to man. God is faithful, and he will not let you be tempted beyond your ability, but with the temptation he will also provide the way of escape, that you may be able to endure it.

1 CORINTHIANS 10:13

My mom is most likely going to read this book, and I'm about to admit something. Maybe she already knows. Who am I kidding? She's a mom; she has probably known the truth for years. Oh well. I have to preface this by saying that I rarely got in trouble as a kid. And I'm not just saying that. It really was rare. I was quiet, and I kind of existed beneath the radar. Besides, my little brother was always so busy getting into trouble that I didn't even have to try hard to remain unnoticed.

There was this one time, though . . . I was a teenager. I can't remember exactly how old, and I can't even remember what I did wrong. Not surprising, since I can hardly remember what I did yesterday. All I know for sure at the time of this writing is that I was not allowed to go on the internet to email my boyfriend (who is now my husband). This was in the early 2000s . . . maybe 2004 or 2005. So cell phones were a thing, but smartphones weren't. I didn't even have a regular old flip phone, and our internet was still dial-up. It really was the good ol' days.

My mom wasn't going to be home when I got home from school, so she must have unplugged the internet before she left, intuitively knowing that I would try to defy her and email my boyfriend (how right she was). She massively underestimated my capabilities, though, because I discovered her little trick and plugged that sucker back in . . . and emailed my boyfriend.

I still feel bad about it to this day. I'm not the kind of girl who disrespects her parents. But I was tempted, and I gave in. There were many ways out of this temptation. My mom tried to provide a way out by unplugging the internet, but I was so determined to have my own way that nothing else mattered to me.

God is such a patient God. He knows how we struggle with sin, which is why He always provides a way out when we're tempted. Thankfully, my indiscretion was small, but the truth is, our daughters are going to be faced with so many temptations and many of them won't be this small. We need to prepare them for this reality, assure them that as God forgives, so do we, and encourage them to always look for a way out of temptation.

Because God is gracious and there's always a way out.

LET'S REFLECT

- Can you think of a time in your life when you let temptation get the better of you?
- Thinking back on that time, can you see where God tried to provide a way out for you?

TAKE ACTION: Make note of this passage today. The next time your daughter is tempted or gives in to temptation, read it with her, and reassure her with the fact that God always provides a way out. Encourage her to always have her eyes open to look for those exits. Importantly, remind her about grace and forgiveness as well.

LET'S PRAY

God, I thank You that You know me so well. You know my weaknesses, and You've provided buffers for me. Continue to strengthen me against temptation, and please help me raise my daughters to be strong against temptation as well. May we always see Your grace in every situation. Amen.

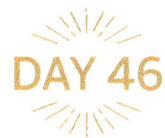

DAY 46

Our Refuge, Our Strength, Our Safety . . . Our God

God is our refuge and strength, a very present help in trouble. Therefore we will not fear though the earth gives way, though the mountains be moved into the heart of the sea, though its waters roar and foam, though the mountains tremble at its swelling.

PSALM 46:1-3

I've mentioned before that my son was really sick with pneumonia in early 2020. Just a couple of short months after he recovered, my brother was hospitalized with what looked like a cancerous tumor. He was in excruciating pain and was hospitalized for weeks while waiting for surgery, all while his wife and five kids were left with a giant question mark over the future of their family.

The year 2020 was difficult for a lot of people, and our family was definitely not an exception to that. But God is so gracious, and He works in us even in the middle of our battles. When the earth gives way and it feels as if the mountains are crashing into the sea, He reminds us that He is our refuge and strength.

Our family received so much prayer in those first few months of 2020, and we truly knew, even in the middle of the storm, that God was our refuge and strength. It became so apparent that He was the only one who could deliver us. Psalm 46 and 91 were a huge comfort to our family during those months, and I ended up writing a song during that time based on those psalms.

The song is called "You Alone." Verse 2 and then into the chorus says, "When sickness comes, and my feet find the snare; when the world turns to terror, and my fears come to life . . . You alone are my refuge, my safety, my God; You alone are right beside me; the rescue is near; You trample the lion, You're crushing the serpent, You alone are my refuge, my safety, my God."

God is sovereign, and He is faithful. Even when the unthinkable happens, His faithfulness can remove our fear. When inconceivable tragedy strikes, His faithfulness brings strength. You are a mom raising a daughter. You will face fear. You will face doubt. You will face things that threaten to break your heart. So will your daughter, and that truth can be hard to swallow.

But you are not alone. When the mountains crumble into the sea and when the earth gives way, know that God is there. He is your refuge, your strength, your safety, your God.

LET'S REFLECT

- What is a struggle you are facing right now?
- Do you find it hard to trust God in the middle of the storms of life?

TAKE ACTION: Today, read Psalms 46 and 91. Let them be an encouragement to you. Whether you're facing peace or trials right now, allow these psalms to remind you of God's faithfulness. If you want to hear the song I referenced today, you can find it on my Instagram @cecily.dickey in the IGTV uploads.

LET'S PRAY

God, I thank You that You are the God of faithful promises. Thank You that You are bigger than this earth and the problems that I face here. Thank You for Your Holy Spirit that is like rivers of living water that bring confidence in any circumstance. Continue to refine and strengthen me, and help me be a picture of Your love and faithfulness for my daughters' watching eyes. Amen.

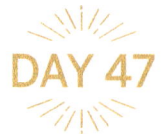

DAY 47

Put Off and Put On

To put off your old self, which belongs to your former manner of life and is corrupt through deceitful desires, and to be renewed in the spirit of your minds, and to put on the new self, created after the likeness of God in true righteousness and holiness.

EPHESIANS 4:22–24

When we meet Christ and embrace Him as Lord, we have to put some things off and put some other things on. Broadly speaking, we put off the old self and put on the new self. The old self is who we were and what we were prone to before we knew the Lord. The new self is the one growing more and more into the likeness of God. The new self should be renewed and refined into truth, righteousness, and holiness.

To be authentic, genuine, positive examples of Christian women for our daughters, we need to make sure we stick with the new self *always* and leave the old self behind permanently. Unfortunately, putting on the new self isn't as simple as saying a prayer (that's only the start). That's why it's difficult to make sure that the old self stays away. It's a process that we must walk through for our entire Christian life.

Our daughters are keen observers. They notice if we put on our new self when we walk into church and allow our old self to rule the roost when we're at home in our comfort zone. We don't want our daughters to think that "Christian" is just a label we slap on before we leave the house. We want our daughters to see that we intentionally choose to be a Christ-follower every day. This means that every day we must put on the new self.

Every morning I take off my nightgown and intentionally choose what clothes I'm going to put on. I "put off" my nightclothes and "put on" my day clothes. In the same way, each day we should be intentionally choosing to put on our new self. The new self is created after the likeness of God. The new self speaks the truth, doesn't let the sun go down on our anger, works hard and honestly, and is generous. The new self is not bitter or wrathful. The new self is kind, tender-hearted, and forgiving (Ephesians 4:25–32).

Put off the old self. Put on the new.

LET'S REFLECT

- What are some characteristics of the old self that are hardest to rid yourself of?
- Which characteristics of the new self are most difficult to cling to?

TAKE ACTION: Each day when you get changed, use it as a reminder to think of how you are to put off the old self and put on the new self. As you do this, remind yourself of the Christ-like characteristics that make up the new self.

LET'S PRAY

Father, I thank You for Your patience with my refinement. I thank You that You don't expect perfection but instead expect a willing and humble heart. I pray that You would transform me more and more into Your likeness each day, as I consistently put on the new self. I pray that through this, You will help me be a positive example of a godly woman for my daughters. Amen.

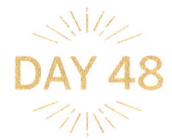

DAY 48

Imitators of God

Therefore be imitators of God, as beloved children. And walk in love, as Christ loved us and gave himself up for us, a fragrant offering and sacrifice to God.

EPHESIANS 5:1–2

My son imitates my husband. Every day he can be found following my husband around, helping with chores, playing basketball with him, talking with him, and listening to him. Our son has a way of acting—we call it man-mode—when he's imitating my husband. He tries to talk like him, look like him, joke like him. He's a *little* man doing his best not just to be a *big* man but to be his dad.

It's totally adorable to watch them interact every day, and I'm so grateful that my son has a great father to emulate. As amazing as my husband is, though, he's not God. He's just a really, really good man. My son works hard at imitating him because he loves him. He follows him and tries to be like him because he appreciates him and admires him.

If my son can follow after another human being that closely, how much more closely should we be following after God? God is perfect. He has no faults. He has perfect justice. He is the perfect Creator. He is the source of all truth . . . and He is offering himself to us. He's asking us to follow Him. He even went so far as to send a piece of the Trinity to Earth, to live a perfect life marked by love, to die for the sins of the world, and to rise and defeat death.

Just as my kids are the beloved children of me and my husband, we're also beloved children of God. Jesus walked on Earth to show us what it looked like to live a life that was filled with love for God and people. As mothers, we also need to live lives of love.

The only way to know how to do that is to imitate our Father in heaven and His Son, Jesus.

LET'S REFLECT

- What resonated with you most from today's reading?
- Whom do you know who has been an incredible example of imitating God in their life?

TAKE ACTION: Commit to reading the Bible and praying each day. To imitate the Lord, you need to know Him.

LET'S PRAY

God, I thank You for who You are. I thank You that You are a good Father who cares for His children. I thank You that You have shown us what it looks like to live a life marked by love. I pray that You will help me be more like You in the life I live and in the love I give. I pray that my daughters would be blessed by my closeness to You. Amen.

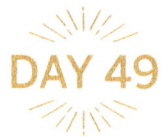

DAY 49

Deserve Is a Dirty Word

Only fear the Lord and serve him faithfully with all your heart. For consider what great things he has done for you.

1 SAMUEL 12:24

This morning, my husband was busy outside in the fields, and I was in the house getting some work done. I knew there was a lot to be done that day, and I knew my kids were capable of helping. I filled up a laundry basket with clean clothes and plopped it on the living room floor so that the kids could work together and get everything folded.

They worked at it together without complaint, and soon the whole basket was folded. My daughter came up to me after and said, "Now I think we really deserve a special snack." It was snack time, so I was happy to give them something to eat; however, I'm always bothered by the word "deserve." That word is a trap.

What do any of us really *deserve*? I can honestly say that God has been more than gracious with me. He has given me more than I physically need. He has provided me with a strong family and community. But most of all, He saved me. He saw me, someone who has sinned, and called me to Himself. He revealed Himself to me, cleansed me from my sin, and gave me a new life. What of that did I deserve? Nothing. But He gave it to me anyway.

I don't want to take all of that grace for granted, and I don't want to raise my kids to take that grace for granted, either. When we live with an expectation that God and the world owe us something, we set ourselves up for bitterness and disappointment. But when we live our lives from a place of thankfulness, everything is seen as grace.

Look at your life. Consider what great things the Lord has done for you. Many are tempted to take the good and simply expect more of it. Instead, though, accept the good that God has offered with a thankful and humble heart, and from that same heart, serve your family. Show your daughter what it looks like to live in awareness of the grace you've been given.

LET'S REFLECT

- Do you ever take the time to reflect on the good things God has done for you?
- Compare and contrast what life is like living with a thankful heart to what life is like living with an entitled one.

TAKE ACTION: Today, make a list of the good things God has done in your life. Remind yourself that those things are gifts, not things that you're entitled to.

LET'S PRAY

Lord, You are so generous. You saw me, someone who has sinned, picked me up, washed me off, and made me pure. I see that my breath and my very life are a gift. I pray that You would help me serve You, my family, and my daughters well—not out of obligation but out of a thankful heart. Amen.

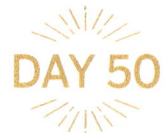

DAY 50

God's Plans Are Always Better

*Commit your work to the Lord, and
your plans will be established.*

PROVERBS 16:3

Hitting all the baby milestones: check. Preschool: check. Elementary school: check. High school: check. University: check. Stable career: check. Happy family: check.

Raising daughters can be overwhelming. All around us, the world is shouting that our babies should be hitting their milestones on time, and preferably early. We should be getting our toddlers on preschool waiting lists years in advance—preferably before they're born (yikes). Elementary school should be marked by advanced reading, and in high school, we should see them making the honor roll and figuring out what they want to do next. University should be focused, and it should set them up well for that stable career that will pay well and afford a bright future. Then comes the happy marriage and the baby in the baby carriage.

This is what the world says we should be grooming our children for. But something is missing on that giant checklist, and it's a big thing. It's an acknowledgment of the fact that raising our daughters is not about us, and it's not about them. Raising our daughters is about raising up people who serve the Lord. That might hit the ears funny in this very "me"-centered world. But none of this is about us, and it's not just about how much or how little our kids succeed.

True parenting success in a Christian worldview means raising kids who know God, love God, serve God, and understand that they are born to be disciples who make more disciples. We should be committing the work we do in parenting to the Lord. All the earthly plans we make mean nothing if our kids don't grow up to acknowledge the One who created them.

I've said it before, and I'll keep saying it. Our goal as mothers should be to raise daughters who know the Lord, love the Lord, and serve the Lord. If that happens, everything else, in the grand scheme of eternity, will be okay. That is my firm and unwavering belief.

LET'S REFLECT

- Are the loud voices of the world's expectations distracting in your parenting journey?
- How would you define success in parenting?

TAKE ACTION: Write today's verse out on a sticky note, and hang it in a prominent place. Let it serve as a reminder that the plans of the Lord are worth so much more than the plans of men and women.

LET'S PRAY

God, I thank You for who You are. I pray that You will speak louder than the world. May I hear You above all competing noise as I seek to raise my daughters. I pray that they will grow to know You, love You, and serve You. I pray that You will fill me with the peace that comes from knowing that my life and the lives of my daughters belong to You. Amen.

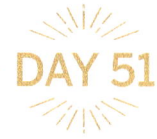

DAY 51

Truth over Lies

If your law had not been my delight, I would have perished in my affliction. I will never forget your precepts, for by them you have given me life.

PSALM 119:92-93

Just because someone says something, that doesn't make it true. This is something I repeat to my kids almost every day. Just today, my son colored a picture of a mallard duck. He's super into birds. My daughter looked at it and said that it didn't look anything like a duck. That wasn't true at all, as it was clearly a duck . . . I could even tell it was a male mallard (my son's obsession with birds has made me an expert on things I never asked to be an expert on).

My son got upset and quickly disparaged *her* picture. She was coloring a picture of some characters from a TV show. He told her it looked nothing like them, and just like that, they were both upset. They each said something untrue about the other and simultaneously believed the untrue thing the other said. This led to me repeating that oft-quoted line: just because someone says something, that doesn't make it true.

As our daughters grow, they are going to hear so many things that are not true. They're going to see messaging that says they have to look a certain way, act a certain way . . . even believe a certain way. That pressure and those lies become an affliction that could easily claim the hearts and souls of our daughters. So, the question is . . . how do we counter that? When we're not standing right beside our daughters to remind them that "just because someone says something, that doesn't make it true," how will they know?

The answer is God. The answer is His Word. Every day, we need to be working toward the goal of planting the gospel so firmly in our daughters' hearts that it is immovable. Our prayer and our ambition should be that no matter the lies thrown at them, no matter what falsehoods try to grow their insecurity, they would clearly see the truth, because the truth is what gives them life.

LET'S REFLECT

- What are the words you use to reassure your daughter of truth?
- What is one way that you can help plant a little truth in your daughter's life today?

TAKE ACTION: Today, remind your daughter of who she is in God's eyes, and read Psalm 139 to her.

LET'S PRAY

God, thank You for being the steady source of truth in this world filled with lies. I pray that You will grow Your Word inside my daughters' hearts so that they will remember the truth even when I'm not beside them. I thank You that You are with them, even when I can't be. Amen.

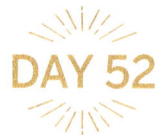

DAY 52

Approval That Matters

For am I now seeking the approval of man, or of God? Or am I trying to please man? If I were still trying to please man, I would not be a servant of Christ.

GALATIANS 1:10

We're going into our fourth year of homeschooling our kids. They started in "regular" school, but a few years ago, we felt strongly that God was calling us to educate our kids at home. At the time, I knew very few people who were homeschooled, and I thought it wasn't a "normal" thing to do.

When we informed our school that we would be pulling the kids out, word started to spread quickly among the parents at school. When people would ask me about it, I made up all sorts of weird excuses for why we were doing it. But my main argument was that the small private school we had them in was too expensive, and we just didn't want to pay for it anymore. That, my friends, was a lie.

Why would I lie like that? The reason I would lie is because I was so worried about what people would think of us if they knew the real reasons. I was worried that if they knew that we felt God had called us to it, they'd think we were misguided. I was worried that they'd think I thought I had better ideas about education than they did. I was worried that they'd see the heart behind our decision and then judge me if I failed at the whole homeschool thing.

Essentially, I feared the opinion of my peers and community. I knew with everything in me that God had called us to do this thing that felt so scary and unusual . . . but I was, for some reason, ashamed to admit that He was the only cause behind our decision to homeschool. Even in my obedience to God's call, I placed the opinions of people over the approval of God. That really made for half-hearted obedience.

I've gotten over my worries about what people think when it comes to homeschooling, but other things still worry me. The same is likely true for you. But God appointed YOU to be your daughter's mother. He is working in you and speaking to you and desiring you would seek after Him with your whole heart as you raise your daughter.

Today, I encourage you to make sure that the voice you value above all others is the voice of God. Today, I encourage you to make sure that the approval you value over all others is the approval of God.

LET'S REFLECT

- Do you struggle to silence the opinions of others as you seek to raise your daughter?
- What judgements are personally most difficult for you to face?

TAKE ACTION: Write down the things you worry most about being judged for, and then take those things to God in prayer.

LET'S PRAY

God, I thank You for this life You've given me. Thank You for trusting me to raise my daughters. I pray that You would silence the critical voices surrounding me and raise up the voices that support and uphold Your truth. Teach me to value Your approval over all others. Amen.

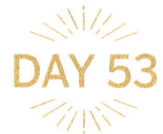

DAY 53

The God Who Sees

So she called the name of the Lord who spoke to her, "You are a God of seeing," for she said, "Truly here I have seen him who looks after me."

GENESIS 16:13

The story of Sarai and Hagar has always made me feel a lot of things. For me, with my modern, Western lens, it's such an impossible scenario to imagine. Sarai hadn't been able to conceive at this point, so she "gave" her servant, Hagar, to Abram in the hope that Hagar would conceive a child *for* them. If that wasn't bad enough, Sarai began to treat Hagar harshly after she conceived, and Hagar ran away.

Hagar was mistreated and felt she had no choice but to run away. She was a woman pregnant and on her own. Sarai's contempt and Abram's indifference were in stark contrast to how God treated Hagar. God sent an angel to her, and God assigned the angel to bless her. God made a promise to Hagar and promised a future for her and her son.

While the people surrounding Hagar were treating her poorly, God was showering her with mercy. Hagar recognized this. Even though she was on the run, God found her. Because of this, she called God "a God of Seeing." She saw that He not only found her, but He cared for her.

This is a truth you will want your daughter to know. She will undoubtedly face hardship and perhaps even rejection. Two things could happen: The first is that she could be devastated and be made to feel worthless. The second (and better) thing that could happen is that she would know that she has a God who sees her and cares for her.

As moms, we want to do all we can to make our daughters feel safe and loved, and we should do everything we can to ensure those things. However, they will not always be under our protection. They need to know the One who is their constant protector. They need to know the God who sees.

LET'S REFLECT

- Has there been a time in your life when you have felt like Hagar?
- In that moment, what did it feel like to go from rejection to redemption?

TAKE ACTION: Today, remind your daughter that God is always watching her. Remind her that He not only sees her, but He cares for her.

LET'S PRAY

Father, I thank You that You are the God who sees us. You see us when we rejoice, and You see us when we suffer. You see us at the top of the mountain and in the valley bottom. Thank You for never ceasing to love us. I pray that my daughters will always see the God who sees them. Amen.

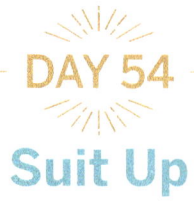

DAY 54

Suit Up

Finally, be strong in the Lord and in the strength of his might. Put on the whole armor of God, that you may be able to stand against the schemes of the devil.

EPHESIANS 6:10–11

My daughter has this little costume that is basically the girl version of Batman. Batgirl, I guess. It's black and gold, and the skirt is black tulle like a ballet tutu. This morning, she was wearing a regular outfit, shorts and a T-shirt. But as I was removing some laundry from the laundry room, she caught a glimpse of her Batgirl costume and asked me to pass it to her.

She put it on over the top of her clothes, and she was transformed. She went from pink shorts and a white shirt to black and gold. But it wasn't just her outfit that was transformed; it was also her persona. As soon as she had the costume on, she smiled with assurance and twirled with confidence. She then strutted up the stairs to show her brothers.

I smiled as I watched her. It is so interesting how an outfit can completely change a person's confidence. Kind of like how back in high school you'd break out your best new outfit for the first day of school. It helps kick up the confidence. When you suit up, for some reason it's easier to stand up.

If this is true about a simple Batgirl costume or a first day of school outfit, how much more true is it for the armor of God? The armor of God consists of a few key pieces: the belt of truth, the breastplate of righteousness, the boots of the gospel of peace, the shield of faith, the helmet of salvation, and the sword of the spirit. If we believe God and focus on the promises He has fulfilled and the promises He still holds, we will feel so confident putting on His armor.

When we suit up with the armor of God and teach our daughters to do the same, there is nothing that can defeat our confidence and our strength. Our confidence and strength will not falter, because their source is God, the Creator of all things.

LET'S REFLECT

- Do you give more thought to your daily outfits than to whether or not you're suiting up with the armor of God?
- Imagine sending your daughter out into the world with the full armor of God. Does that thought give you confidence as her mother?

TAKE ACTION: Discuss the armor of God with your daughter. If she's still young enough, play dress-up with her. Have her dress as a superhero, and ask whether it makes her feel strong. Then explain to her how much stronger she will be with the armor of God.

LET'S PRAY

Thank You, Lord, for the armor You have provided. Life can be rough; it can wear us down and make us weak and tired. Thank You for offering us Your strength. I pray that my daughters will grow to depend on You and that they will grow in confidence as they learn to suit up with Your armor. Amen.

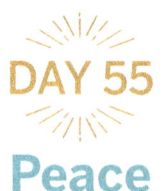

DAY 55

Peace

Peace I leave with you; my peace I give to you. Not as the world gives do I give to you. Let not your hearts be troubled, neither let them be afraid.

JOHN 14:27

I want you to think about the last year of your life. Consider the events that have happened around the world and the things you have personally encountered. How much peace has the world offered you? I actually believe the world has tried to steal my peace.

With so much bad news being broadcast it's easy to understand why feelings of fear and anxiety are high right now. The effects of this are felt everywhere—at schools, in stores, at church, and sometimes even amid our own families. But Jesus has a different way.

We want our daughters to live in peace. Of course, we are realistic, and we know that our girls live in a world that will never be perfect. But Jesus offers them (and us) the kind of peace that is not dependent on our circumstances.

In today's passage, Jesus is speaking with his disciples. He's giving them instruction ahead of His crucifixion and ascension. At this time, the disciples still don't fully understand what Jesus is about to endure and that His time on Earth will soon be completed (for a while, anyway). Jesus and the disciples are heading into circumstances of anguish rather than peace.

Jesus's disciples didn't want Him to leave the earth. But even though violence was being waged against Jesus and His disciples, He was assuring them of the peace He was giving them. Jesus promised them—and He promises all those who trust in Him—the Holy Spirit, the Helper, the Giver of peace.

What assurance this is for us, mothers raising daughters! The world may never be a utopia, but that doesn't mean our daughters can't know peace. The news headlines may claim the sky is falling, but as long as our daughters hold fast to Jesus through the power of the Holy Spirit, peace will never be absent from them.

LET'S REFLECT

- Have you felt your peace slipping away from you due to recent world events?
- How can you help ensure that your daughter will live a life that is filled with peace?

TAKE ACTION: Be real with your daughter today. Talk about something going on in the world that could easily steal peace, but then show her that true peace cannot be taken away from her.

LET'S PRAY

Thank You, Father of peace. I need You every moment of every day as I seek to cling to You and Your peace in a world that seems bent against peace. I pray that You will help me guide my daughters in Your ways and into Your peace. Amen.

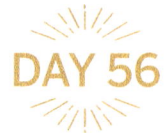

DAY 56

Give Your Fear to the Lord

*I sought the Lord, and he answered me and
delivered me from all my fears.*

PSALM 34:4

Fear. It can make a person do some crazy things. On a rainy April day a few years ago, I put my baby girl down for a nap and turned on a show for my two-year-old and four-year-old so that I could go outside to water my seedlings in the greenhouse. At that point in my life, alone time was rare and beautiful, so I was completely delighted to head out to the warmth of the greenhouse, smell the soil, and listen to the rain patter gently on the plastic.

After I finished watering, I turned to leave the greenhouse and pushed at the door. It wouldn't open. I pushed harder, and it still wouldn't move. At this point, panic began creeping in. As all moms do, I began to imagine worst-case scenarios. Despite all logic, I became convinced that a serial killer/kidnapper had locked me in the greenhouse and then run to the house to take my kids. With that horrible thought firmly in my sleep-deprived brain, I backed up to the end of the greenhouse and ran forward, flinging my whole body at the door. It wouldn't open.

This continued for quite some time, but it became apparent I couldn't get out. I phoned everyone who would be nearby, but no one answered their phones. With my panic only growing instead of receding, I phoned the police. I couldn't get out, and no one else was around to help me.

Soon, I heard the officer outside the greenhouse, and he opened the door. Before he said anything to me, he reached around the door jamb and pulled a string. It was just a latch, and all I had to do was pull the string. I had no idea that was on my own greenhouse. I was humiliated and soon realized that even without the handy string latch, I could have sliced my way out of the soft, plastic greenhouse with the pointy end of a watering can. Oh well. Hindsight is 20-20 and all that.

Fear is a God-given emotion that helps keep us safe. But like all emotions, it shouldn't run us. That day, I let it run me . . . and it ran me nowhere good. As a mom raising a daughter, you're also going to feel fear. Use it as the gift God intended it to be. Use it with logic, and use it with faith. Seek wisdom, and give your fear to the Lord; let Him deliver you from your fear. Because if you're anything like me . . . you really need Him.

LET'S REFLECT

- Describe a time when fear drove you to do something that didn't make any sense.
- Do you find it difficult to give your fears to God? Why or why not?

TAKE ACTION: Find a way to remind yourself to seek God when you're fearful. Perhaps you could post this Bible verse somewhere or order it as a print for your wall. Find a way to make sure that God is in charge of your fear, rather than you.

LET'S PRAY

Thank You that You are God. Thank You that You listen and don't leave me alone in my fear. I pray that You would surround me with Your peace and wisdom as I raise my daughters and help them grow into women who find their security in You as well. Amen.

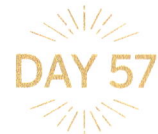

DAY 57

Using the Bad for the Good

And now do not be distressed or angry with yourselves because you sold me here, for God sent me before you to preserve life. For the famine has been in the land these two years, and there are yet five years in which there will be neither plowing nor harvest. And God sent me before you to preserve for you a remnant on earth, and to keep alive for you many survivors. So it was not you who sent me here, but God.

GENESIS 45:5–8

Often, it seems many of us think that the bad things we go through in life are because God doesn't care. This story flips that presupposition on its head to show us the truth.

Joseph had been sold into slavery by his jealous brothers (awful), but when he got to Egypt, he became a successful man. He was in the home of Potiphar, who was captain of the guard and an officer of Pharaoh. It was going well for Joseph there until Potiphar's wife began to make a move on Joseph. Joseph turned her down, and she lied and told her husband that Joseph had tried to take advantage of her. Because of this, Joseph was thrown in prison.

So first, his family sold him into slavery, and second, he was thrown in prison because someone lied about him. Those are both terrible and horrific life events. While in prison, though, Joseph met a couple of guys who had some wild dreams. Joseph was able to interpret them correctly, and he asked one of them to put in a good word for him with Pharaoh when he was released. The man forgot, though, leaving Joseph in prison.

One day, though, Pharaoh had a wild dream about fat cows and skinny cows, and the man remembered that Joseph was able to interpret dreams. Joseph was let out of prison to interpret Pharaoh's dream. Joseph interpreted it correctly, and Pharaoh put

Joseph in a position of great honor. Joseph had the responsibility of rationing food before a coming famine. His brothers came to Egypt to find food, and Joseph revealed that he was still alive and very powerful.

Joseph could have been angry at them, but God helped him see that He used all the bad things that happened in Joseph's life for *good*. Joseph saved Egypt and his own family from famine. This allowed Joseph to be an integral part of God's plan for His people.

As mothers, we have the important job of teaching our daughters that God uses EVERY event in life for the good of those who love Him (Romans 8:28). We need to teach our daughters that this won't mean constant sunshine and rainbows, but that God remembers us, values us, and has so much good in store for us . . . Just like He did for Joseph.

LET'S REFLECT

- What resonated the most with you from today's reading?
- When you go through hard times, are you tempted to think God doesn't care? If so, how does the story of Joseph change that?

TAKE ACTION: Today, reflect on some of the hard things you've been through, and see whether you can identify how God was working through it all. Take note of those things to share with your daughter when she faces her own struggles.

LET'S PRAY

God, I thank You that You have a bigger perspective than I do. Thank You for not wasting the bad things we experience in life but using them for good. You have shown me that there is always a reason for hope, and I'm so grateful for that. Amen.

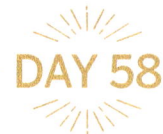

DAY 58

Every Good and Perfect Gift

Every good gift and every perfect gift is from above, coming down from the Father of lights, with whom there is no variation or shadow due to change.

JAMES 1:17

The creation story describes how God spoke light into existence; made the heavens and the water; spoke plants into being; formed the sun, moon, and stars; and filled the oceans with life and the earth with animals. The creation story then tells us how God created man and woman in His image. He breathed life into them, and Genesis 1:28 says, "And God blessed them."

God blessed Adam and Eve at the very beginning, even though He knew they would fall. He blessed every generation that followed them, and He has blessed you and your daughter, too.

The creation story does a beautiful job of showing us that there would be nothing here if not for God. Everything we see around us is a gift from our heavenly Father. When my kids were born, I was in awe when I heard them make their first cry. I cried when I saw their faces for the first time. And when their little hands wrapped around my finger, well, just that small action was like watching a miracle unfold. They hadn't yet done much, but it was so clear to me that their very existence was a gift.

As time goes on and as life gets busy, it can be easy for us to let our blessings become burdens. When that happens, we need to stop and re-evaluate. We need to go back to the beginning. We need to strip back all the unnecessary trappings that we tend to put into our lives and see what God has done. He made you. He saved you through his Son, Jesus. He gave you a daughter. He made you a mother. He breathed life into your child.

The food you eat is because God created. The oxygen you breathe is because God created. The home you live in is because God created. And the child you're raising belongs first to the Lord. Your life is a gift. The things you have are a gift. And your daughter is a gift that was entrusted to you by her heavenly Father.

Every good and perfect gift in your life is from God. That makes every day Thanksgiving.

LET'S REFLECT

- Do you find it hard to be thankful? Why or why not?
- How would it affect your motherhood if you took the time to see all the good that God has gifted you?

TAKE ACTION: Today, make a list of the things you clearly see as gifts from God. Say a prayer of thanks for each one.

LET'S PRAY

God, I thank You for being so generous. I pray that You'll open my eyes to see all the beautiful things You have surrounded me with. I pray that I would grow in thankfulness each day and that my thankful heart would serve as a catalyst for my daughters' hearts to grow in thankfulness as well. Amen.

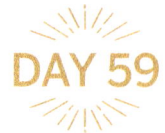

DAY 59

Worship as a Way of Life

Therefore let us be grateful for receiving a kingdom that cannot be shaken, and thus let us offer to God acceptable worship, with reverence and awe, for our God is a consuming fire.

HEBREWS 12:28-29

I love to listen to my daughter pray. She prays like she's talking to a friend. She prays eagerly and with her heart full of thankfulness. She prays on her own and with her family. She never says no to prayer, and she always does it with an open heart.

I also love to watch her worship. During church, she splits her time between giggling with friends and taking some time to sing. At home, though, she pours her heart into her worship. She sings with passion, even coming up with her own lyrics and melodies on the spot. She sings to God whatever is on her heart and mind in a given moment.

The way she worships is in contrast to how adults often worship. As a worship leader, I've observed many stoic adults while we sing to the Lord. Now, worship isn't only singing on a Sunday. Worship can be accomplished in all aspects of our lives—the way we work, the way we play, the way we raise our families and interact with our coworkers. Worship is declaring the greatness of God and responding in a way that aligns with His greatness.

Once, Jesus's disciples tried to stop people from bringing children to Him. Jesus responded by saying, "Truly, I say to you, whoever does not receive the kingdom of God like a child shall not enter it" (Luke 18:17). Jesus talks about *receiving* the kingdom like a child. If we *truly* believe the gospel and *receive* Christ, shouldn't our worship reflect that? My daughter's worship does, but I'm not so sure mine always does.

Now, lest you think my sweet girl is perfect after I described her worship and prayer habits, I think it's important I tell you what she said the other day. She was misbehaving and not helping her brothers clean up. I said to her that God didn't make her lazy and rude but kind and helpful. She looked at me calmly, shrugged her shoulders, and said, "I'm not so sure about that."

She's not perfect, but she has a heart that beats for the Lord. As mothers who believe the gospel, we should have hearts that do the same. Let's live lives that are marked with worship that is filled with reverence, awe, and thankfulness.

LET'S REFLECT

- Do you find it difficult to worship in the way God calls us to? Why or why not?
- Do you ever worship with your daughter? If so, what is that like?

TAKE ACTION: Today, put on some worship music, and worship with your daughter. Begin to make a habit of it.

LET'S PRAY

God, Your grace is so evident in my life. Because of this, I pour out thankful worship to You. I pray that You would continually remind me of Your greatness, so that I live a life that reflects that. I pray that You would help me receive Your kingdom like a child and that my daughters would come to know You and worship You as well. Amen.

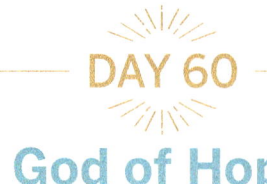

DAY 60

God of Hope

May the God of hope fill you with all joy and peace in believing, so that by the power of the Holy Spirit you may abound in hope.

ROMANS 15:13

Today is Day 60. We've come a long way together, and I want to leave you with a benediction. A benediction is a blessing. I write a lot of benedictions for our church, and I love doing it. But as much as I love writing benedictions, the ones that are already in the Word of God can't be beaten.

You are a mother. You are raising an amazing girl to be a strong, capable, and faith-filled woman. Along the way, you are going to face challenges, be struck with fear, and wonder whether you're cut out to do the hard work of raising a human. You will inevitably have days that suck and leave you feeling weaker than when you woke up that morning. But those days won't break you.

Those days won't break you, because you serve the God of hope. He has been faithful from the first day of creation until now. He sent His Son so hope could even exist. The God of hope doesn't expect you will have everything figured out, but the God of hope will fill you with the joy and peace that come from believing the gospel. And on the days when it's hard to believe, ask Him to help your unbelief (Mark 9:24).

Remember you have the Holy Spirit living in you—the same Spirit that raised Christ Jesus from the dead (Romans 8:11). If that Spirit can bring the dead to life, imagine what it can do in you and your daughter.

Raising daughters may not be for the faint of heart, but when you do grow faint, remember that the Lord carries you on wings like eagles (Isaiah 40:31). When you feel alone, remember that God will never leave you or forsake you (Deuteronomy 31:8). When you feel fearful, remember that God gave you a spirit of power and love and self-control (2 Timothy 1:7).

God does not make mistakes. He chose you to be the mother to your daughter, and He entrusted His precious child to you. Let truth fill you with awe, and may it drive you forward in all that you do.

As we bring this devotional to a close, I want to pray this blessing over you: "May the God of hope fill you with all joy and peace in believing, so that by the power of the Holy Spirit you may abound in hope" (Romans 15:13). Amen.

LET'S REFLECT

- Over the past 60 days, what did God reveal to you?
- Are you ready to live your life and raise your daughter while being fully dependent on the God of hope?

TAKE ACTION: Today, read through all the Bible verses cited in today's devotion. Let them serve to bring you closer to the God of hope.

LET'S PRAY

God, You are so good. You provide hope in a dark and uncertain world. You provide hope for me, someone who has sinned. You washed me clean and allowed me to serve You and raise my daughters. I pray that I would keep my eyes fixed on You and that my daughters would see my heart truly transforming, more and more each day, into Your image. I ask this in the precious name of Jesus, Your Son. Amen.

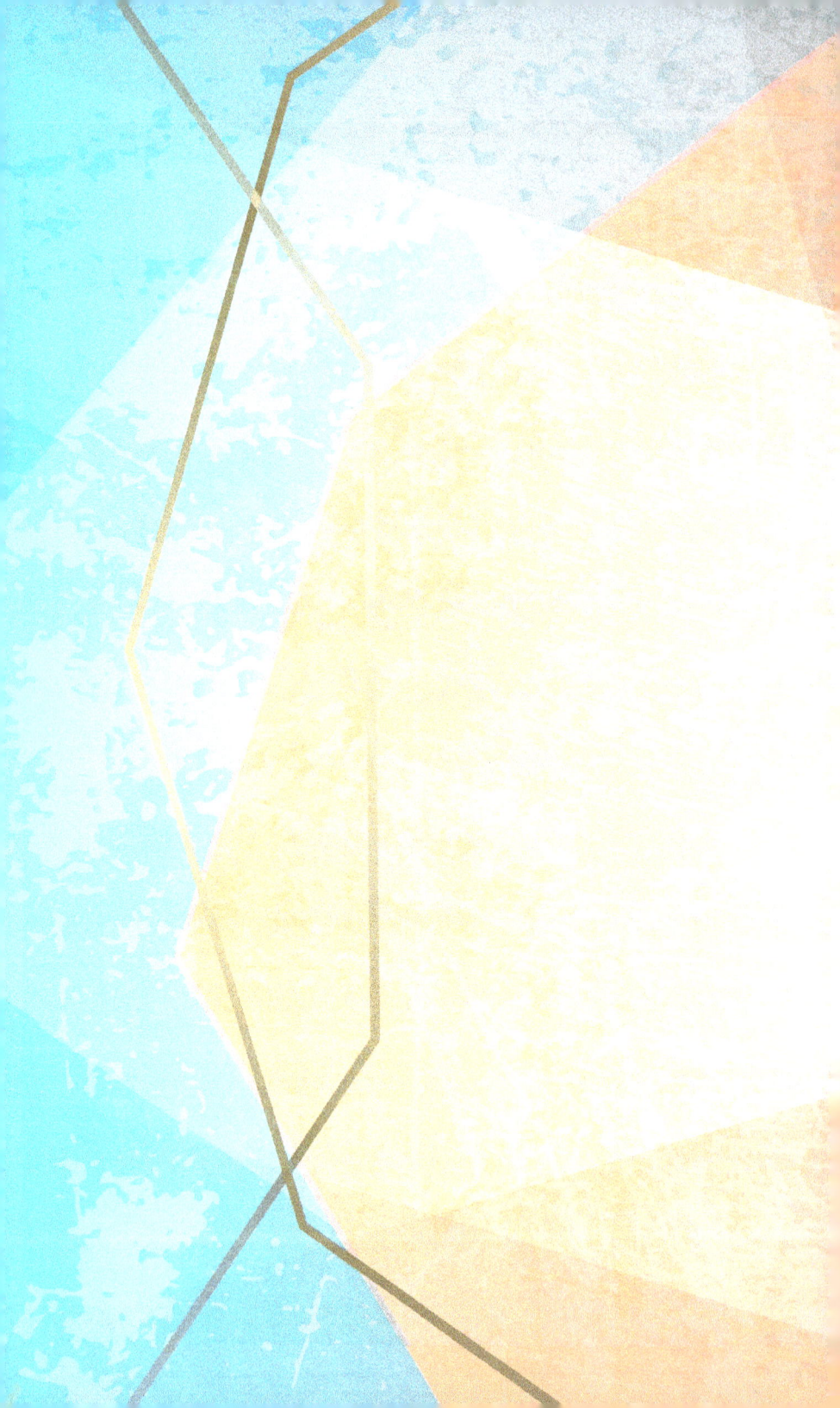

A FINAL WORD

You made it to the end of our 60-day adventure together! I pray that this book helped draw you closer to your daughter and to the Lord.

Raising daughters is a gift, a privilege, and a challenge. As you continue to mother your daughter, remember that God uses all the good and all the bad to refine you more and more into His image. Remember that the world will try to distract you and your daughter from the ultimate goal of serving the Lord. Because of this, you need to intentionally hold fast to God and His Word.

Remember, also, that God doesn't send you out and leave you alone. He has sent you a Helper, the Holy Spirit. That Spirit is the same one who raised Christ Jesus from the dead. It is not a spirit of fear, but of power, love, and self-control. When you are weak, He is strong.

God bless, mama. May you raise your daughter to be like an arrow in the hand of a warrior as you serve alongside her in the building up of the kingdom of God.

Acknowledgments

Writing this book was an adventure that wouldn't have been possible without my husband. Thank you, Kyle, for supporting me and keeping the kids happy and entertained. I will always insist that I married the best man in the world, and if anyone disagrees with me about that, they're just plain wrong.

Thank you, kids, for your patience with me. While I was writing, I only saw your fingers creeping under my door a handful of times, and the constant somersaults and giggles I heard on the other side of the wall kept me entertained.

Mom and Gramma, you two ladies were so helpful to me as I worked on this book. You allowed my kids to show up at your door for jelly beans and a chat, you helped me harvest and process our garden produce, and you were unfailingly encouraging. I love you both. Thank you for teaching me how to be a mom.

Thank you to Rockridge Press, Callisto Media, and Matt Buonaguoro for seeking me out and taking a chance on me. Thank you to Carolyn Abate for being such a fantastic editor. You were so encouraging and supportive throughout the whole process.

Most of all, thank You, Lord. Without You, I really wouldn't have much to say. This book exists because of You.

About the Author

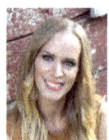

CECILY DICKEY lives in British Columbia, Canada. She is a wife and mom, worship leader, writer, and cohost of *The Boom Clap Podcast*. Follow her on Instagram at @cecily.dickey.

www.ingramcontent.com/pod-product-compliance
Lightning Source LLC
LaVergne TN
LVHW010308070426
835510LV00025B/3409